Mediterranean Diet

**Including Mediterranean diet recipes
and a review of Mediterranean food
and healthy lifestyle**

Elisabetta Parisi

First Printing, 2013

ISBN - 13:978-1484800218

ISBN - 10:1484800214

Printed in the United States of America

Dedication

For Alan

Mediterranean Diet

**Including Mediterranean diet recipes
and a review of Mediterranean food
and healthy lifestyle**

Table of Contents

Introduction

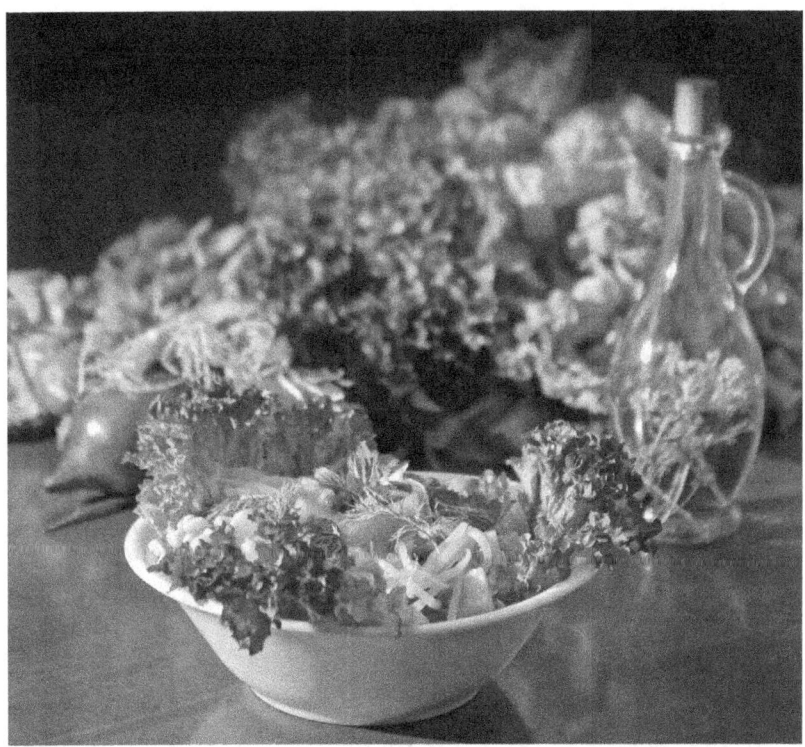

Mediterranean diets are based on the food eaten by the coastal dwellers of countries such as Greece, Italy and Spain. The food that these people eat depends very much on the local environment. As a result olives and olive oil are very important as are fresh fish caught from the Mediterranean Sea. Add to this, whole foods such as local green vegetables, fruits, whole grain cereals and nuts then you have the essence of the diet that is eaten. Also included in this diet is the moderate consumption of alcohol, often in the form of red wine.

The rest of the world is interested in Mediterranean food because of the health benefits that the people, living in these regions, seem to get from eating it. The diet is just as important for the things that either aren't consumed or are eaten in only small amounts. As a result people in these regions tend to eat only small amounts of red meat, processed meat, dairy products and sweet foods.

The Mediterranean diet has never been as popular in news reporting as it is these days. Interest has steadily increased since it was reported to us in 2005 that a scientific study showed that people following a Mediterranean style diet tended to live longer. In recent times interest has greatly increased, especially since it was reported in October 2012 that the majority of people living on the Greek island of Ikaria lived to a very old age. In fact they are two and a half times more likely to live until they are ninety compared to American people. In addition to this longevity, the people of Ikaria are also more likely to have an active and useful old age. In contrast, in North Western countries such as the USA, old age is more associated with having health problems and having to be cared for in an old people's home. It is therefore no wonder that scientists and doctors are keen to work out what the secret to this long and active life involves. Scientific studies have continued to be produced and the latest one published in February 2013 showed that people on a Mediterranean diet were significantly less likely to suffer from heart attacks and strokes compared to people that are even on ordinary low fat diets.

The aim of this book is to consider the evidence from these studies and reports and then to detail how you can implement to best aspects of a Mediterranean diet for yourself.

The Secrets of Ikaria

In an article in The New York Times magazine written by Dan Buettner the life of the Ikarian people was examined in order to try and identify the reasons why so many people lived such active lives well into the elderly years. The research wasn't totally scientific, in that it just tried to catch a flavour of what was actually going on in Ikaria to allow people to live so long. It was also felt that the resulting effects weren't just caused by their diet alone. It was thought that it was as much to do with the general lifestyle that they followed in combination with the food that they ate.

Ikaria is a small Greek island just off the coast of Turkey. It is only about one hundred square miles in size and currently has around ten thousand Greek inhabitants. It has a ridge of mountains with cliffs that come straight out of the sea and has many steep hills. It has some hot thermal springs which have been part of the island's attraction as a health resort for something around two and a half thousand years.

Here are some of the things that were thought to be important in order to get the full benefits of a Mediterranean lifestyle:

They wake up late and go to bed late. They tend to wake up naturally and then take things as they come through the day. They aren't ruled by clocks and watches. In fact, they don't wear watches, and clocks on the island rarely work or show the correct time. This in turn leads to a reduction in stress levels both at work and home, compared to the rest of the Western world. You only have to think about the stress of arriving late in normal Western cultures. Late lunch and lots of naps all result in a relaxed atmosphere. Taking naps on a regular basis is thought to be able to reduce the risk of coronary heart disease by up to forty percent especially if they are taken at least three times a week.

Their diet centres on virgin olive oil, wild legumes, milk from goats, wine and even coffee. In addition to this they consume in the region of six times the amount of bean type foods such as lentils and chickpeas compared to people in America.

It is also important to consider the things that they don't eat or eat in small quantities. They consume only a little sugar, white flour and meat. This in turn means that they eat very little as far as saturated fats are concerned. They don't eat any processed food. This is important because it has recently been noted in the UK press that processed food could be causing as many as one in thirty deaths. Nobody is sure why this is, but it is thought that preservatives such as nitrates and the plastic packaging wrapping many supermarket foods may play a role in this. The Ikarians have eliminated this factor entirely by only eating fresh food that they grow or rear themselves. The greens that they grow in gardens and fields on the island are fresh and therefore contain more nutrients compared with those that lie on supermarket shelves for days or even weeks on end. In addition to this, these freshly grown vegetables will have far lower amounts of pesticides in and on them compared to the greens eaten in America and other Northern countries of the Western world.

A typical basic Ikarian diet for a day would be as follows:

Breakfast
A drink of herb tea, homemade wine, goat's milk or coffee together with local honey and whole grain bread.

Lunch
Beans such as Lentils, black eyed peas and chick peas, potatoes and legumes such as dandelion, fennel and a wild spinach greens. Added to this are garden grown greens that are in season at the time.

Supper
Herbal teas and homemade wine with family and friends who visit just after sunset.

Dinner
This usually consists of whole grain bread with goat's milk

In general it has been found that Ikarians eat about 6 times the amount of beans a day compared to the average American. Fish is consumed at least 2 times a week and meat only 5 times in a month. A lot of olive oil and olives are also consumed. Olive oil may be used in cooking and also served with the local bread. In terms of wine consumption it was found that up to 4 glasses may be consumed each day.

Local honey is also important. It is used to treat a number of different medical problems including influenza and wounds. Older people also tend to start their day with a spoonful of honey. This is looked upon as a medicine. It has been determined by scientists that honey contains a number of antimicrobial agents. Honey has been used in the treatment of wounds and other illnesses for thousands of years.

Meat from such things as the family reared pig would be kept for special occasions such as festivals including Christmas and Easter when it would be slaughtered and used for the festival and some months after this. This would be consumed in small amounts over the time as larded pork.

The Ikarians make and drink a variety of different local mountain teas. These are made from the many herbs that grow naturally on the island. The dried herbs are steeped in boiled water to make the teas. The kinds of herbs used to make teas include wild sage, marjoram and rosemary. There is a special kind of mint tea and another one using dandelion leaves together with lemon. These teas are often enjoyed at the end of the day as a soothing and warming drink. They are often considered by the locals to be of medicinal use when they drink them.

The benefits of their diet can be seen by examining the individual components. They have only a small amount of saturated fat from dairy and meat. This is of course associated with reducing the problems caused by heart and vascular disease. The olive oil that they consume has the effect of increasing good cholesterol in the blood and at the same time cutting down the levels of bad cholesterol. This is especially the case when the oil is taken cold rather than in a heated form. Mediterranean diets often have olive oil consumed by dipping bread in it. Goat's milk is easily digested by older people and contains the essential amino acid called Tryptophan which has the effect of increasing serotonin levels in the brain which increases people's feelings of well being. The wild greens that they use in their meals contain high levels of antioxidants which can help to reduce ageing of the body's cells. The wine that is consumed is good as part of a Mediterranean diet plan because it helps the body to take in more flavenoid antioxidants from the digesting food as it sits in the gut. Coffee is thought to be responsible for helping to reduce diabetes and heart disease. The bread which is often a locally made type of sour dough is thought to help in the reduction of blood sugar levels after meals. This in turn also helps to prevent diabetes from occurring because blood sugar levels are more easily maintained at the correct levels. The rest of the vegetables including locally grown potatoes add valuable minerals, vitamins and fibre.

Regular exercise also plays a part in their lifestyle. This includes gardening and other manual work that has to be done on the island. Getting about the island is done by walking and because of the steep nature of the hills there, people can end up walking up and down many hills each day. It is impossible to get away from this exercise if you are going to lead a normal life and visit friends and neighbours each day. It is typical for Ikarians to visit their neighbours or friends in the evening and drink homemade wine and tea. The Ikarians also tend to keep busy and get involved in the community and the households of their extended families even after they have been retired for many years. This is in great contrast to other western countries where people who retire can end up doing very little. This has been linked to early death. You only have to think of those friends and relatives who retire and then end up dying within just a few weeks, months or years. The retired on the island also claim to have healthy sex lives. Those individuals between sixty five and one hundred appear to continue to have sex on a regular basis. This all adds to the continued activity and healthy lifestyles enjoyed by the islanders no matter what age that they are

The specific benefits of the Ikarian diet and lifestyle mean that the islanders can live up to 10 years longer than the rest of us before they have to deal with such conditions as heart disease and cancer. Rates of depression are also reduced. The diet also reduces the number of people that go onto suffer from Alzheimer's. This again is important because the numbers of people suffering from Alzheimer's in the rest of the world is very troubling. Old people on Ikaria are in general far more physically and mentally active until a greater age compared to people from America and the rest of the Western world.

The Ikarians are in a unique position in terms of the diet that they consume compared to the rest of us in other Western countries. This is because of the island's physical situation. In terms of history, the island of Ikaria has been one that has escaped a mass influx of people. This is in part because it has no natural harbours and the steep cliffs in the coastal regions tended to put off, all but the most persistent, visitors in the past. The island has therefore had to be self sufficient and to its benefit it continues to be self sufficient. This means that the island has escaped much of the modernisation that other Greek islands have had to endure. You only have to look at Ikaria's nearest neighbour, the island of Samos. This island has a vast tourist region and houses there now cost huge amounts of money. Money drives the life of the people on Samos. This has meant that all of the trappings of modern life have ended up there. This includes processed food, lack of community and a more modern lifestyle in general. All of these things have passed Ikaria by, and as a result it still depends on a traditional way of life. On Ikaria it is therefore easy to maintain a healthy diet and lifestyle because everybody else is doing it and there are very few temptations from modern processed foods and other lifestyle choices. The lower dependence on money has meant that the Ikarians have managed to maintain their relaxed lifestyle which in turn has contributed to their longer and healthier lives. How much more difficult would it be for the rest of us to take up an

Ikarian lifestyle? We have all of the temptations from processed food, modern agricultural practices, modern lifestyles and, in general, a lack of community to support us. Despite all of these difficulties there are still a lot of things that we can learn from the Ikarians and introducing even some of their, ideas as lifestyle choices, is bound to help us in small ways to get to where we want to be.

The Spanish Trial

The results of the latest study, into the effects of a Mediterranean diet on health, were released in February of 2013 in the New England Journal of Medicine after the study had been running for a total of five years. The article about the study is called ' Primary Prevention of Cardiovascular Disease with a Mediterranean Diet'. The study took place in Spain, which is one of the places where the Mediterranean diet originated. This has been the largest trial involving the Mediterranean diet to date. It involved nearly seven and a half thousand people. People from a range of different locations in Spain were enrolled into the trial. The trial was aimed at men and women who were considered to be at risk from heart disease; however, none of them actually had any form of cardiovascular disease right at the start of the trial. The sorts of people enrolled were either suffering from type two diabetes or any three of the following risk factors: smoking, high blood pressure, high levels of bad LDL cholesterol, low levels of good HDL cholesterol, obesity or a family history of heart problems. In addition to this the selected participants were between the ages of 55 and 80 for men and 60 to 80 for women. There was also an attempt to try and have equal numbers of men and women on the trial.

In the trial the study group were randomly divided into three different groups. Each group was given a different diet to follow. Instruction was given to the subjects and checks were made to try and ensure that the diets were being followed to the best of the subjects' ability. The first group had to follow a Mediterranean diet with added extra virgin olive oil. The second group were asked to follow a Mediterranean diet with added nuts. The third group had to follow a normal reduced fat diet. This third group was the control group so that the other 2 groups could be compared to them. Each group was expected to follow their given diet for the 5 years of the trial.

The basic diet followed by the 2 Mediterranean groups contained at least: 3 servings of fresh fruit per day, 2 servings of fresh vegetables per day, 3 servings of fatty fish and other sea foods per week, 3 servings of legumes per week and 2 servings of sofrito per week. Sofrito is a fresh sauce that is made by simmering tomatoes, olive oil and onion with herbs and garlic. In addition to this they were also encouraged to switch red meat for white meat and those who normally drank alcohol were encouraged to drink at least 7 glasses of red wine per week. There were a number of food items that they were asked to try and keep to set maximums as part of their Mediterranean diet. They were asked to keep soda drinks to less that 1 per day, spreading fats to less than 1 serving per day, red and processed meats to less that 1 serving per day and bought sweets, baked items and pastries to less than 3 servings per week. The Olive oil group followed the above diet with the addition of having to consume at least 4 tablespoons of extra virgin Polyphenol rich olive oil per day. This olive oil could be used in cooking, salad dressings or taken raw with such things as bread. The nut group consumed at least 3 servings of nuts per week instead of olive oil. The recommended amount of nuts was actually 30g per day, which it was suggested should be made up of half of walnuts and a quarter each of hazelnuts and almonds.

The control group were expected to follow a low fat diet. This was recommended to consist of at least: 3 servings per day of low fat dairy foods, 3 servings per day of bread, pasta, potatoes or rice, 3 servings per day of fresh fruit, 3 servings per week of fish or seafood in general. The people on this diet were also expected to make sure that other particular foods were kept below a particular level. These foods should have been no more than: 2 tablespoons per day of vegetable oil, 1 serving per week of bought pastries and sweets, 1 serving per week of fried snacks and nuts, 1 serving per week of processed meats and red meat, 1 serving per week of fatty fish, 1 serving per week of spreading fats and 2 servings per week of sofrito. In addition to this they were expected to remove any visible fat from meat and soups before eating them.

The three groups were allowed to follow their individual diets for the five year period. There were checks during this time to ensure that everybody was following the correct diet and instruction was given on a regular basis to make sure that they kept to the diet given to them.

The results of the trial involved counting the total number of heart attacks, strokes and deaths caused by heart disease for each of the dietary groups. The results for the olive oil and nut groups were then compared with the low diet control group to see if there were and significant differences. It was found that the olive oil and nut diets led to a reduction of 30 percent in the risk of ending up with cardiovascular problems and strokes compared to the low fat control diet. This is a large reduction in the risk of getting these conditions. It definitely shows that the ordinary low fat diet recommended by many medical professionals doesn't have any benefit when it comes to heart disease and strokes. It is worth noting that the Mediterranean diets used were not restricted in the amount of energy that could be taken in. They are therefore not diets that are concerned with weight loss.

There are a few things that need to be kept in mind when it comes to this Spanish trial. Firstly, all the people involved were Mediterranean in origin and therefore questions have to be asked as to whether the results can be transferred to other ethnic groups. Secondly, all of the people involved were at risk of getting heart and stroke problems and therefore care has to be taken when considering the whole of a population where people aren't at risk from suffering from these. It is thought that the majority of the benefits obtained from the Mediterranean diet were due to the enrichment of them with olive oil and nut content

Where to Start?

Olive oil is central to the Mediterranean diet and so this is a good place to start. Just about everybody will have a bottle of olive oil at the back of their cupboards and the temptation is to just grab that and start using it. This could be a big mistake, because olive oil has a limited shelf life. The longer that olive oil is left lying around the fewer valuable nutrients that it will contain. It only takes around six months for olive oil to become significantly degraded in terms of its nutrient content. If your bottle of olive oil is over a year old then it will contain practically nothing of any use in terms of health giving qualities. You should therefore get rid of these old bottles and go and buy some fresh extra virgin olive oil straight away! When you buy your olive oil it is worth noting that the colour of it has no relation to its quality. The colour is more likely to be due to the local growing conditions and olive trees where the oil is produced so don't worry about it.

Once you have the fresh extra virgin olive oil you can start improving your diet straight away. The first thing that you should do is start to use olive oil where you would be using fats such as butter, saturated oils and any fats like as lard. You can also use olive oil in sauces that you make and with salad. We all like to have things that taste good so a nice idea is to get some quality fresh wholemeal bread, break it into chunks and dip it into olive oil ratter than spreading it with butter or margarine.

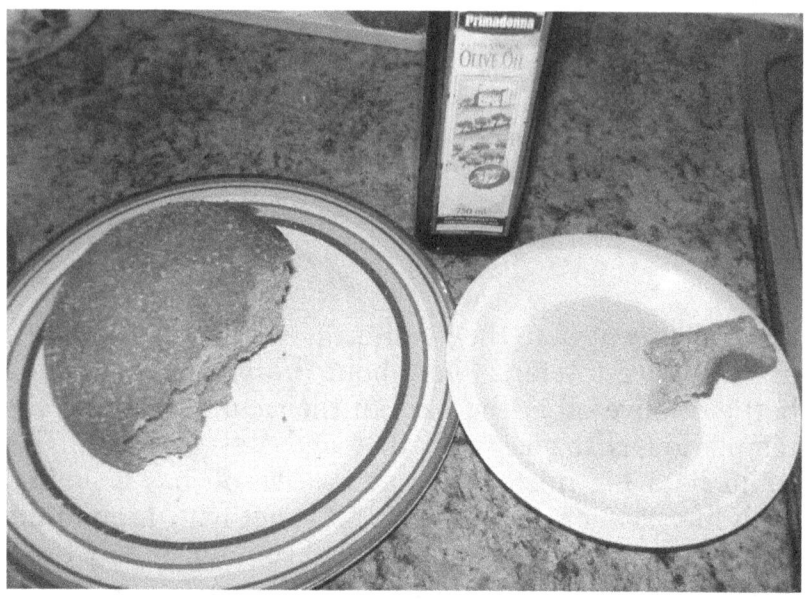

This makes a lovely accompaniment to meals. This is the way that the Spanish serve their meals. There is always fresh bread and a container of olive oil on the table. Once you get a taste for bread with olive oil you will be more likely to have it as a snack rather than salted potato chips, pies or pastries. When you are using olive oil in your cooking you should make sure that you only apply a low or moderate heat to it. If the oil begins to smoke you will be destroying the valuable nutrients in it. If this happens it is best to discard the food you are trying to cook and begin again with fresh oil. You should also remember to keep your bottle of olive oil in a dark and cool place so that it will remain in good form for a longer amount of time. The reason for this is that heat and light speed up the loss of the nutrients in the oil.

Add more tomatoes to your meals. Tomato sauces are used a lot in Mediterranean regions. You only have to think about all of the tomato sauces used by the Italians with their meals. In actual fact they end up eating some form of tomato in their meals just about every day. With tomatoes, cooking actually adds to the valuable nutrients within your meals. Tomatoes contain a powerful antioxidant called lycopene which becomes far more easily absorbed from the digestive system once the tomato has been cooked. It therefore doesn't matter how long you leave your tomato sauces cooking on the stove. Tomatoes also contain other major antioxidants which are known to help in decreasing the risk of cancers especially of the prostate gland and the pancreas.

Wine is another important part of the Mediterranean diet. Red wine is thought to be the best due to it containing important polyphenol compounds which help in protecting the heart. The polyphenols are found in the skins of grapes and are more prominent in red wine because the skins are allowed to be in contact with the fermenting juice during its production. Small amounts of alcohol also help to increase the amount of good cholesterol in the blood stream. Red wine is generally only recommended for those people who already drink alcohol and those who won't be unduly affected by consuming alcohol. It is thought that regular consumption of red wine is best, and only in small amounts. Something like seven small five ounce glasses of red wine spread throughout the week should do the trick.

Start to eat mainly plant type foods such as fruit, vegetables including legumes, whole grains, whole grain rice, pasta and nuts. In Greece people tend to eat at least nine servings of fresh fruit and vegetables per day. These will be rich in antioxidants and this goes towards creating the lower levels of bad cholesterol that are found in people who naturally eat a Mediterranean style diet. Greeks also eat very little red meat and this is another typical trait for people in the Mediterranean areas. As shown by the scientific report in the last chapter nuts are an important part of any Mediterranean diet. Nuts are very high in fat content. Up to eighty percent of the energy content is in actual fact made up of fats. The good news is that these fats are not the saturated kind. Due to this high fat content you shouldn't eat huge amounts of nuts. It is best to keep it to just a handful of nuts per day. You should always make sure that you eat the raw nuts and not those that are salted or have a sugar style coating around them. Examples of good nuts to include in your diet are almonds, cashews, pistachios and walnuts. You can keep nuts near by for use as snacks which will stop you slipping and eating sweets, biscuits or pastries instead. Whole grains could be in the form of breads or pasta. When eating whole grain bread try to get used to the idea of eating it by dipping into extra virgin olive oil. You can also get flavoured Olive oil which can make dipping with bread more interesting. This is the Mediterranean way. You should avoid adding butter or margarines as these contain manufactured trans fats in order to make them spreadable. Trans fats are really bad in terms of adding to your cholesterol problems. If you are looking for something more spreadable then you can try Tahini. This is made with blended sesame seeds. This is also a Mediterranean style food and can be used for dipping with bread as well as olive oil on its own.

As already discussed, olive oil is the main type of fat that you should be consuming. The Mediterranean diet isn't a low fat based diet. Instead of avoiding fats altogether you are expected to make sensible choices about the fats that you consume. You should try to avoid saturated fats and substitute them for sources of food that contain unsaturated fats. This means avoiding those foods such as red meat that are high in saturated fats. Instead of this, you should be eating more fish. Fatty fish are the best sources of this type of fat. Examples of these are such fish as mackerel, trout, herring, sardines, tuna and salmon. Fatty fish contain Omega 3 fatty acids and these can help lower the amount of triglycerides in the blood and makes blood less likely to clot while it is in blood vessels. They also reduce the risk of heart attacks as well as reducing blood pressure and maintaining the health of blood vessels. It is no surprise that the Mediterranean diet is associated with those areas in the South of countries such as Italy, Greece and Spain where fresh fish is in plentiful supply.

The Mediterranean diet isn't necessarily a low salt diet because such things as olives are often preserved in salt and as a result you can't actually avoid it altogether. However, it is best to avoid salt wherever possible because of its effect on blood pressure. As a result, you should not eat nuts that have been salted and you shouldn't use it in a shaker at the table on your meals either. During cooking salt is basically just added as a flavour enhancer, so in order to get round adding salt you should try to make the foods that you cook more flavoursome by adding extra herbs and spices. Herbs and spices are both tasty and full of health giving substances as well. These are therefore 2 good reasons for using them in cooking and when making salads.

You should just make small changes in your diet to start with and then look for interesting Mediterranean foods in stores, restaurants and cookery books in order to increase the range of foods that you can make.

Costs

Compared to the food that you usually make you may find that some of the ingredients used in the Mediterranean diet are a little more expensive. Typically extra virgin olive oil and nuts are quite expensive when you compare them with the alternatives. You shouldn't let this put you off. In terms of olive oil you should shop around. Some of the cut price supermarkets have high quality olive oil at a reduced price. So long as it is extra virgin oil there shouldn't be a problem. You can also think about buying a larger quantity of the oil and save by bulk buying. You should just make sure that you will use the olive oil within 6 months while it is at its best. The same goes for buying nuts. Buy them in bulk or you can also try buying from web sites.

You should also consider the fact that you will be reducing the amount of meat that you eat. Red meat such as beef is an expensive food, so switching to a more vegetarian based diet should save you some money in the long run. Vegetables can also be bought cheaper by going to a local produce market. These are often a lot cheaper when compared to supermarkets. Farmer's markets and farm shops can also be considered when it comes to buying your vegetables. Farm shops often have discounts and deals for buying larger quantities. Instead of buying a few potatoes consider getting a 22 kg bag. So long as you keep your potatoes in the right conditions they should last a reasonable time. The same thing can be achieved by buying nets of carrots and onions. When buying from a farm shop they may have the option of buying washed or dirty versions of the products. Dirty carrots still have some of the soil attached to them and because they haven't been damaged by a washing process they tend to last longer.

In terms of herbs, you can try growing them in your garden or even on the windowsill, if you haven't got a suitable outside space. Herbs are in general quite easy to grow and you can buy seeds for them quite cheaply. Some herbs such as chives, mint and rosemary will continue to grow from one year to the next. You really only have to plant them once. Mint is rather like a weed and once it is planted it will start to appear all over the place. As the years pass by these plants will grow large, take little of your time in care and produce the freshest herbs that you can get.

Cut herbs bought from the market or shop, have quite a limited life and you need to use them within just a few days. An alternative is to buy one of the potted versions from supermarkets. These have become quite popular and so long as you look after them by putting them in a light place, such as a window ledge, and keep them watered will supply you with fresh herbs for a longer amount of time. These potted plants often don't work that well in the winter time due to lack of light and the cold.

Another idea is to freeze the herbs that you don't use on the day. You can chop them and freeze them in portions ready to use. One way to do this is to use an ice cube tray. Put your chopped herbs into the ice compartments with some water and allow them to freeze. Once they have frozen into cubes you can empty them out and put them into labelled plastic bags to be kept in the freezer and used when needed. This can be a real time saver when you have to get meals prepared quickly.

If fresh herbs aren't available you can always use dried versions. These are usually reasonably cheap to buy and have a long shelf life. You can also produce your own dried versions of the herbs that you have. This works best for those herbs that are already quite resilient such as rosemary and thyme. Simply hang the herb branches up in a dry place and allow them to dry over time. Once they are dry you can store them in glass jars for use at a later date. I also dry spare chillies that I buy from the market. I buy a standard amount of the chillies and after using the few that I need on the day I simply leave them in the paper bag that they came in to dry on the windowsill in the kitchen. If your chillies came in a plastic bag you should transfer them to a paper bag before starting to dry them. Every now and then check the chillies in the bag and remove any that have gone mouldy and shake them about a bit so that they all get an equal chance to dry. Once they are dry they will last for many months and you will then get a good return for the small initial investment that you made.

Wine can be another expensive item especially if the country where you live applies a large tax to alcohol products. If your country produces its own wine, it might be an idea to buy the local varieties as they may be a lot cheaper. You can also get wine at a good price from the cheaper supermarkets. You should look for deals where you get the wine cheaper for buying a few bottles or even buying a whole case. It really isn't necessary to get the most expensive wines unless you really have a taste for them and have the money to afford them. Table wines will do the same job so long as they are red wines

Wholemeal bread shouldn't be anymore expensive than white bread. There may be just a small difference in cost. Consider going to a small local bakery or a supermarket that bakes its own bread. It shouldn't cost any more and you will get a quality product that is a joy to eat. You can also try baking your own bread. This would allow you to experiment with different types of bread. You can get bread machines that will do most of the work for you. I have found that it is best to let the machine do all of the mixing work and then bake the actual bread in a real oven. You can experiment with rustic Italian bread and produce some really tasty bread to dip in your extra virgin olive oil.

Mediterranean Diet Recipes

The important thing to keep in mind is that the Mediterranean diet is not about suffering and restricting the amount you eat, as with a lot of diets that are designed for weight loss. The Mediterranean diet is all about enjoying food. You may have to make some different choices about what you eat, but the recipes that you substitute for you old ones have been developed and refined over centuries by the people of the Mediterranean region, making them the tasty dishes that are still enjoyed by millions of people today. Mediterranean food is delicious, so you should be looking forward to experiencing great news meals and great new tastes.

There are a lot of so called Mediterranean recipes out there to choose from but you have to be careful which ones that you use. The reason for this is that there are a number of people who are making up recipes to kind of fit in with the Mediterranean taste. These may also be ones that have been developed for tourists in the region as well. As a result they are often over loaded with meat dishes. Another thing that you will notice is that dairy products such as cheese are often added in abundance to these recipes. I think that this is because they have often been adapted to try and fit in with the normal American style diet. These will then appeal to the unsuspecting who will happily consume lots of red meat and cheese thinking that they are well on their way to a healthy diet. Such recipes won't help you in your quest for a real authentic Mediterranean diet, and you should avoid them. Instead you should try to select those ones that are either vegetarian or fish based without added cream and cheese ingredients.

Look through the ingredients of any recipe first, and check that the essential ingredients are there. These should definitely include lots of olive oil and fresh vegetables. You should also look to see if they contain whole grains as well. If the recipe doesn't quite match up to your expectations you can try putting in some substitutions. Substitute extra virgin olive oil for any other oil, whole grains for refined grains such as; brown rice for white rice, fresh vegetables for canned ones, yoghurt for creams and white meat or fish for red meat. In some cases it will depend on what you can buy in your area and canned items such as red kidney beans are often not a bad item to use. However, where possible use the fresh ingredients. Use fresh herbs wherever possible, but using dried herbs won't be a problem, if they are unavailable or out of season. You should also keep in mind that any substitutions may change the recipe cooking times, and as a result you will need to experiment to get you meal cooked as it should be. In this book I have included a number of basic recipes which will help to get you started in building up a repertoire of good basic Mediterranean foods.

In constructing these recipes I have attempted to reduce the salt content as much as possible. Obviously, adding salt is a personal choice but you should keep in mind that the Wold Health Organization has stated that consuming excess salt is a worldwide problem that can cause high blood pressure and strokes. Personally I don't add salt to any of the foods that I cook. I always just leave it out. This is my choice and I have gotten used to the taste. You may decide to do this for yourself. If you find that the food doesn't taste as pronounced as you would like it to, you should try adding extra herbs and spices such as pepper as well as extra garlic. These can all give extra flavour without the problems that excess salt can cause. You should remember that you are getting sufficient salt already from products that you buy such as Olives, whole meal bread and other everyday products. The salt is added by the manufacturer for either preservation or as a flavour enhancer.

Some cheese in recipes maybe inevitable, but you should make sure that you use it for flavour rather than just for body. The addition of highly flavoured cheeses such as Parmesan is to be expected with some meals but if you find that you can do without it you can certainly leave it out. Cheese is also another source of salt which is always used in its manufacture. When you are selecting recipes for a Mediterranean diet, certainly, make sure that you aren't eating dishes with cheese everyday. Try to be sensible and only use it in some of the meals that you make each week.

Spanish Sofrito

Ingredients

28 ounce can crushed tomatoes
1 long green sweet pepper
1 medium yellow onion
3 large cloves garlic
Extra virgin olive oil
1 tsp sweet paprika
Lemon

Method

Peel the onion and garlic and then finely chop it into small pieces. Chop the green pepper into small pieces of around half a cm in size. Mince the garlic cloves.

Pour a little olive oil into a large frying pan and place on a medium heat. Swirl the oil around to coat the bottom of the pan. Add the chopped onions to the pan and cook them until they become transparent. Make sure that you don't burn them. Next, put the chopped green pepper into the pan and cook while stirring for about another 5 minutes. Make sure that the pepper doesn't burn and turn down the heat and add extra olive oil if you need to.

Add the minced garlic to the pan and cook for a further few minutes. Put the tomatoes into the pan and add the paprika pepper together with a few squeezes of lemon. Stir the contents of the pan until everything is well mixed. Cook on a low to medium heat for a further fifteen minutes. You can keep the sauce in the refrigerator for up to five days.

You can serve the sofrito with rice or eggs or use it as the tomato sauce element in many other dishes such as with wholemeal pasta. You can easily increase the amount of garlic, pepper and spices to suit your individual taste.

Egg and Asparagus salad

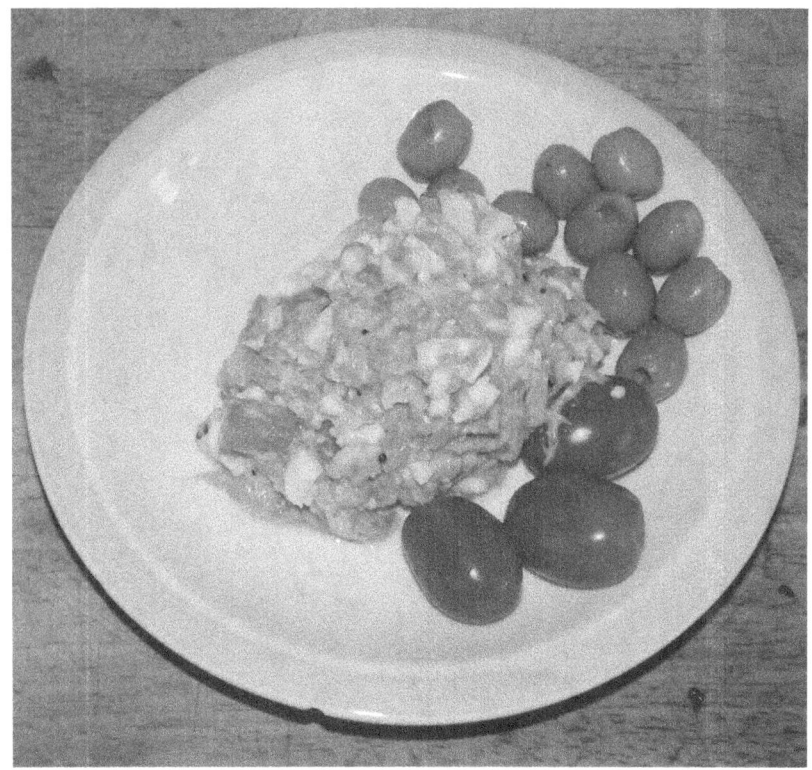

Ingredients

Bunch of asparagus
Extra virgin olive oil
2 eggs
Red wine vinegar
Salt and pepper

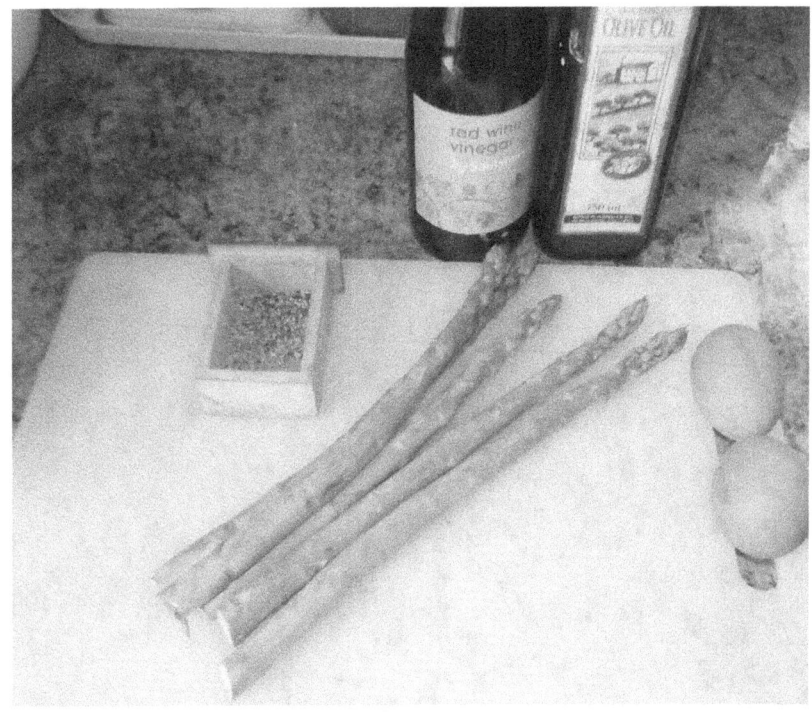

Method

Boil the eggs in a pan of water until they are hard boiled. Remove the tough ends of the Asparagus and boil the rest of the asparagus shoots until they are nice and tender. Drain off the water and allow both the asparagus and the eggs to cool back down to room temperature.

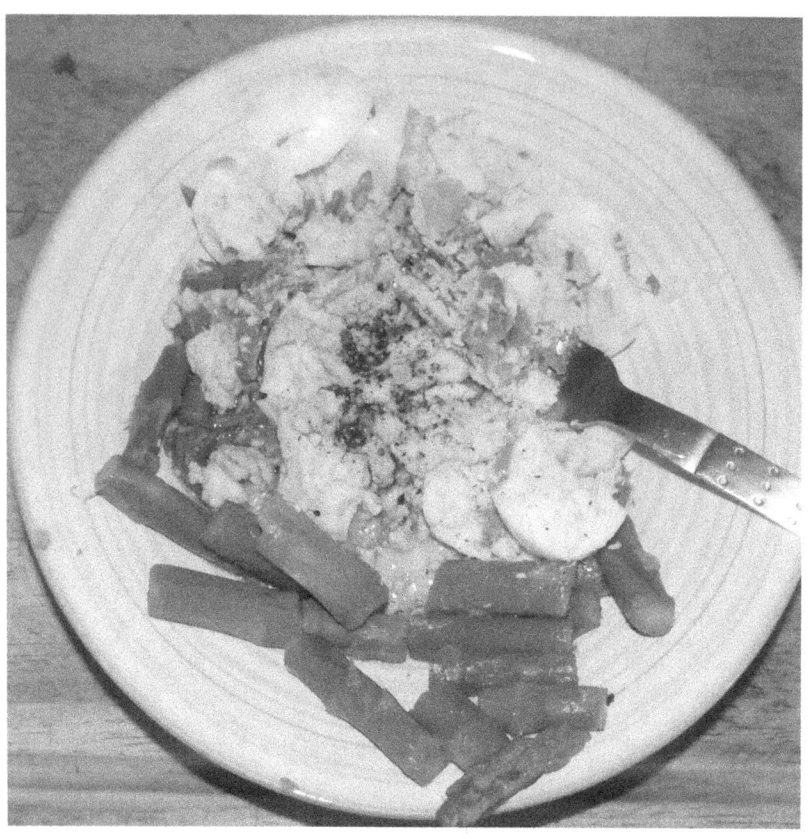

Peel the hard boiled eggs and mash them together with the asparagus. Continue to mash while adding some olive oil, red wine vinegar, salt and pepper to taste.

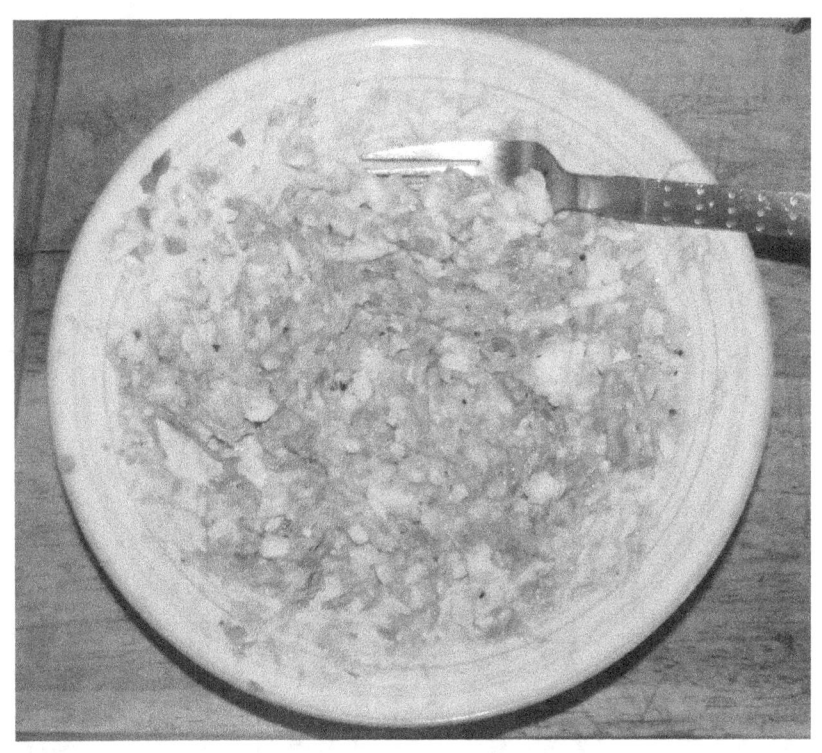

Mashed egg and asparagus mixture before serving

Salad with red kidney beans

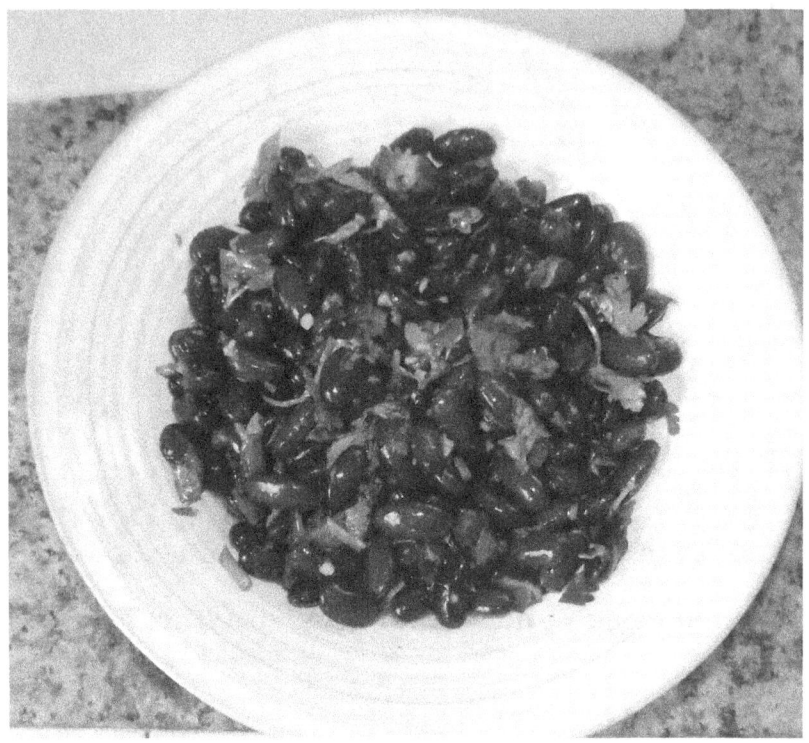

Ingredients

1 can of red kidney beans
2 clove garlic
2 tbsp chopped parsley
2 tbsp extra virgin olive oil
1 tbsp red wine vinegar
Salt
Pepper

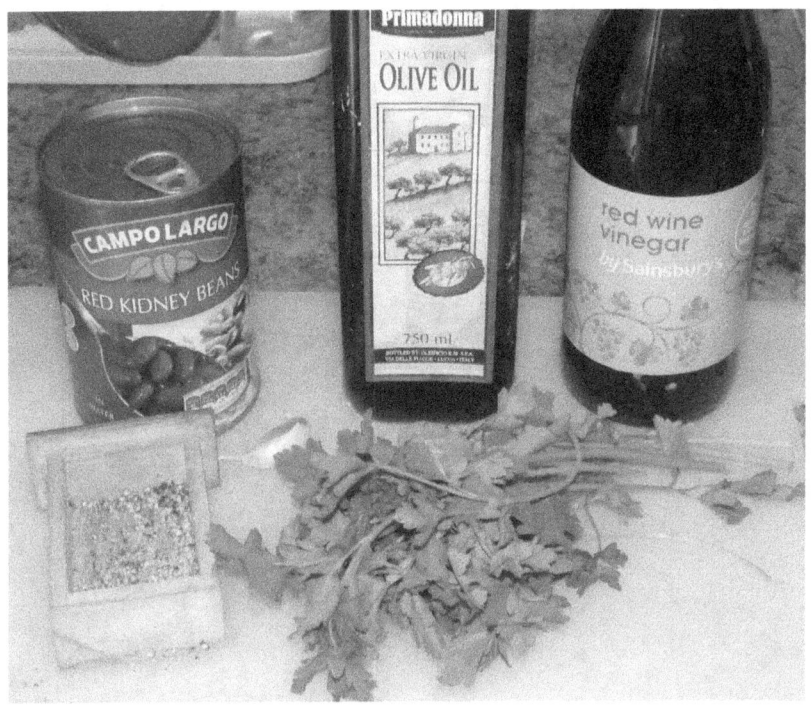

Method

Empty and drain the can of red kidney beans and put them into a mixing bowl. Mince the garlic and add this together with the chopped parsley to the bowl. Add the olive oil, red wine vinegar salt and pepper to taste.

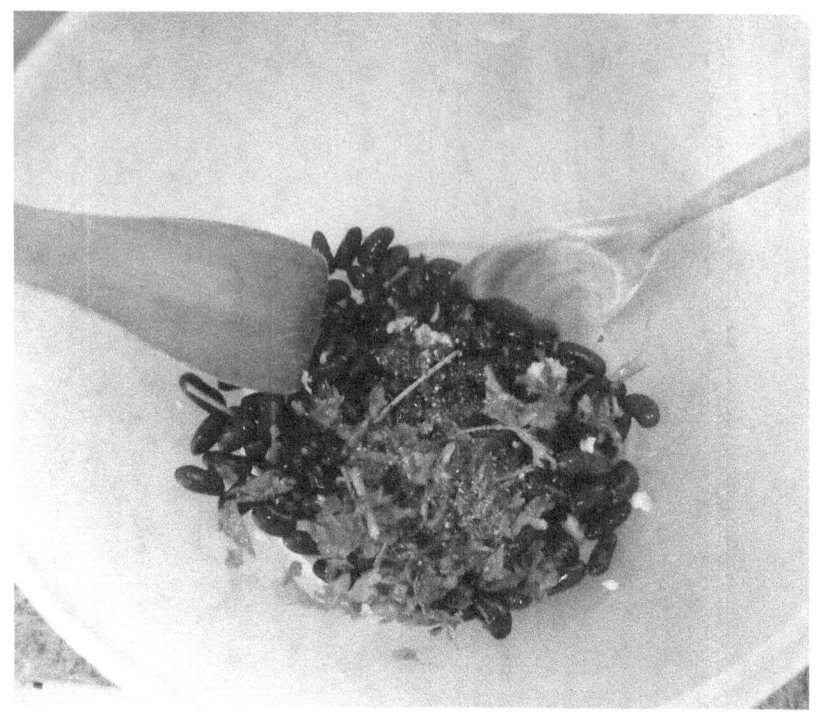

Toss the salad to combine the ingredients and serve.

Gazpacho

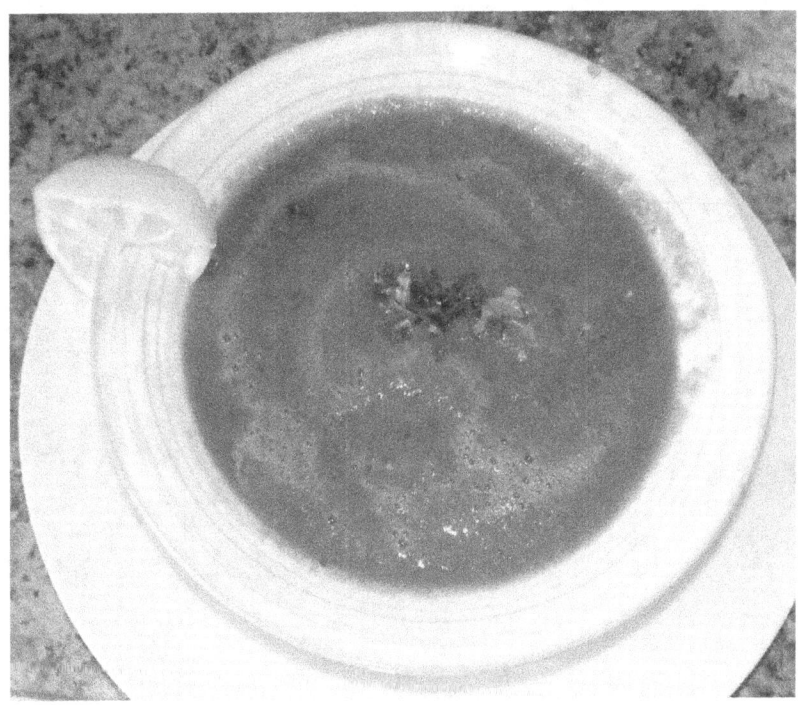

Ingredients

3 medium sized tomatoes
1 cucumber
1 red bell pepper
1 medium onion
3 cups tomato juice
2 tablespoons chopped fresh mixed herbs
3 tbsp red wine vinegar
2 cloves garlic
2 tablespoons tomato paste
1/2 lemon
Course ground sea salt

Cayenne pepper

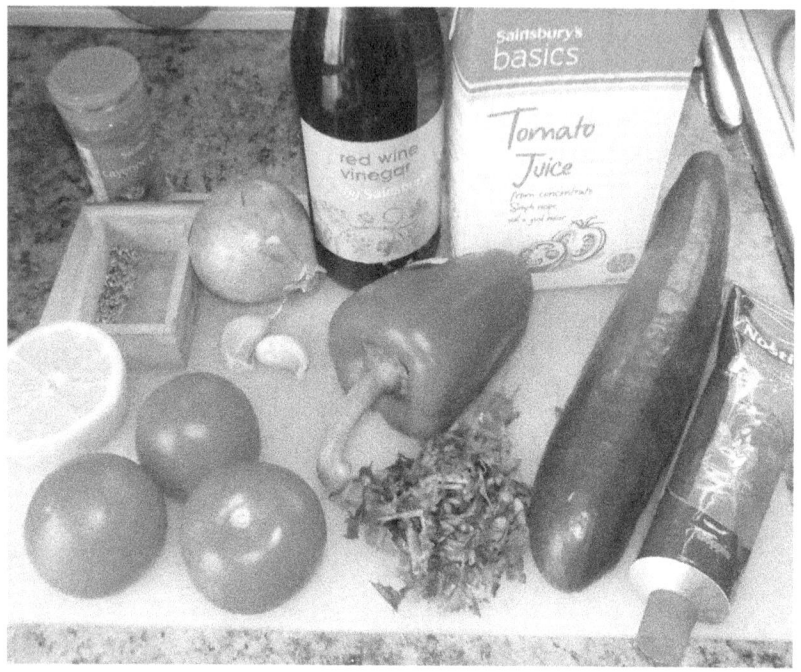

Method

Chop the tomatoes and the cucumber. Chop the red pepper and the onion. Peel and finely chop the garlic. Squeeze the juice from the half lemon and put into a small bowl.

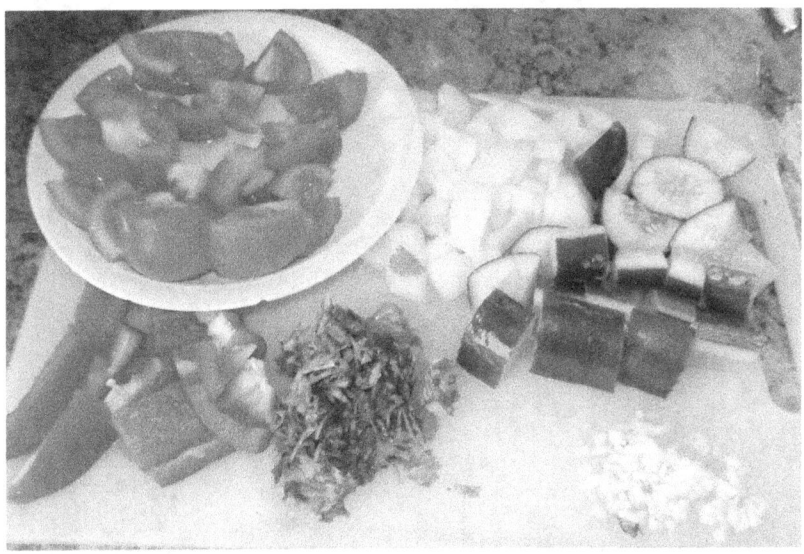

Put the tomatoes, cucumber, red pepper, onion, garlic, tomato juice, mixed herbs, tomato paste and red wine vinegar into a blender or food processor.

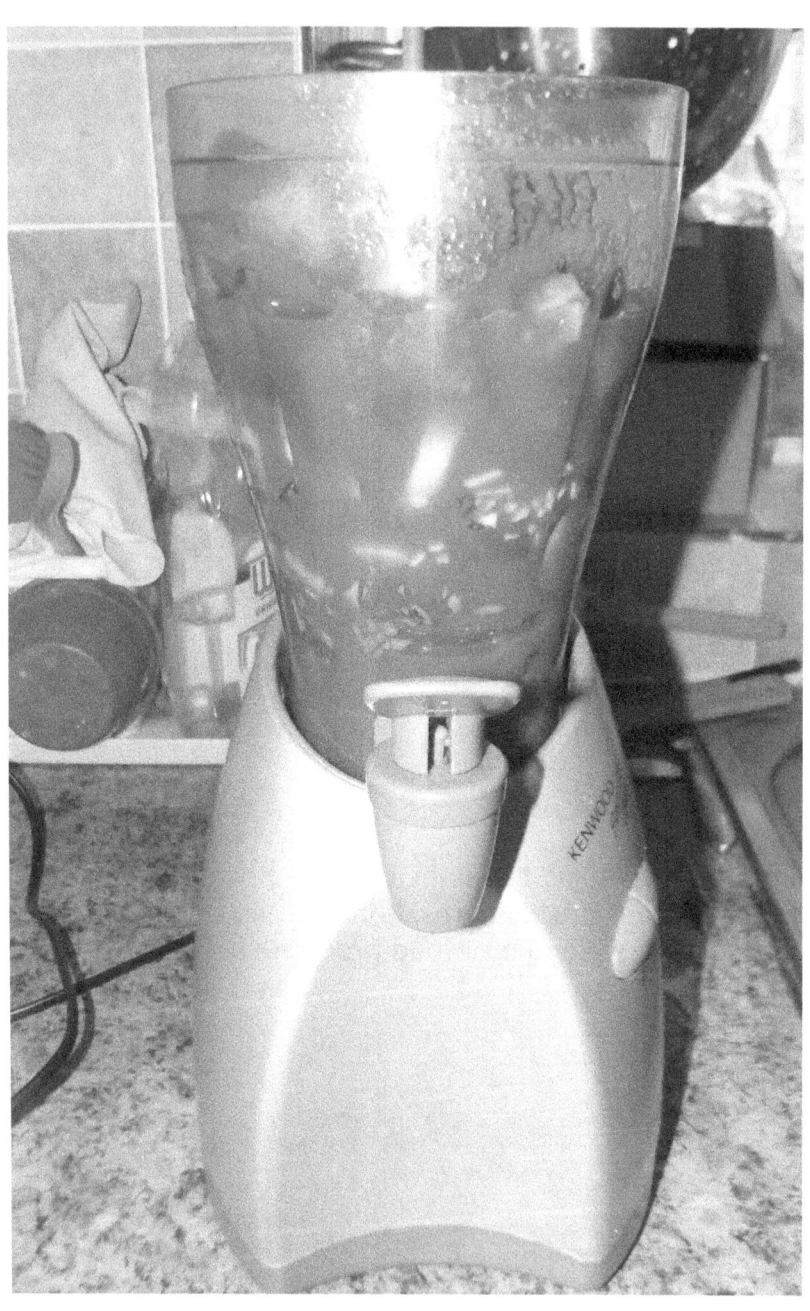

Puree the mixture until it is nice and smooth.

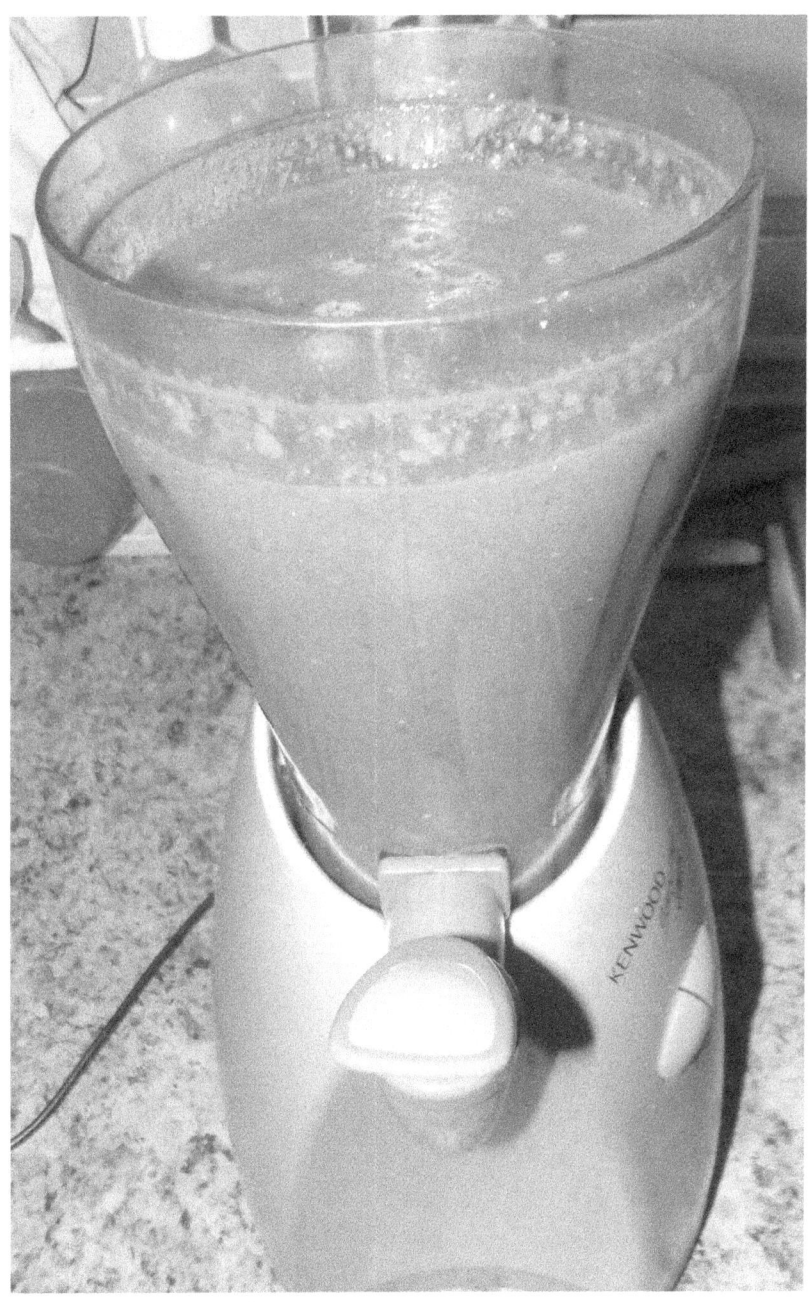

Season the mixture with sea salt, cayenne pepper and lemon juice to get the taste that you like. Put the

Gazpacho into a covered bowl and place in the refrigerator to chill for a few hours before serving with chunks of fresh whole grain bread and olive oil for dipping.

To make a smoother Gazpacho you can peel the tomatoes, remove the seeds and then chop them. You can do the same with the cucumber by removing the seeds and chopping it. I usually leave them in as they are so that it adds to the rustic feel of this wonderful food. You can also cut back or increase the amount of red wine vinegar depending on your personal preference.

Potato salad

Ingredients

1 tbsp extra virgin olive oil
1 small onion
1 garlic clove
1 tsp chopped fresh oregano
200g cherry tomatoes
1 small red pepper
300g small new potatoes
25g black olives
Handful of fresh basil leaves
Salt and pepper seasoning

Method

Thinly slice the onion. Crush the garlic clove. Slice the black olives. Roughly tear the basil leaves. Peel the tomatoes.

Put the potatoes into a pan of boiling water and cook for about 15 minutes until they are tender.

Put the olive oil into a saucepan and heat it on a medium/low heat. Add the onion and gently cook until it is nice and soft. Add the garlic and oregano and cook for about a further minute. Add the tomatoes and pepper and season with salt and pepper to taste. Cook gently for about another 10 minutes.

Drain the potatoes and mix them with the sauce in the other pan. Serve the potato salad while it is still warm and garnish each serving with the basil and the sliced olives.

Salmon with tomatoes and olives

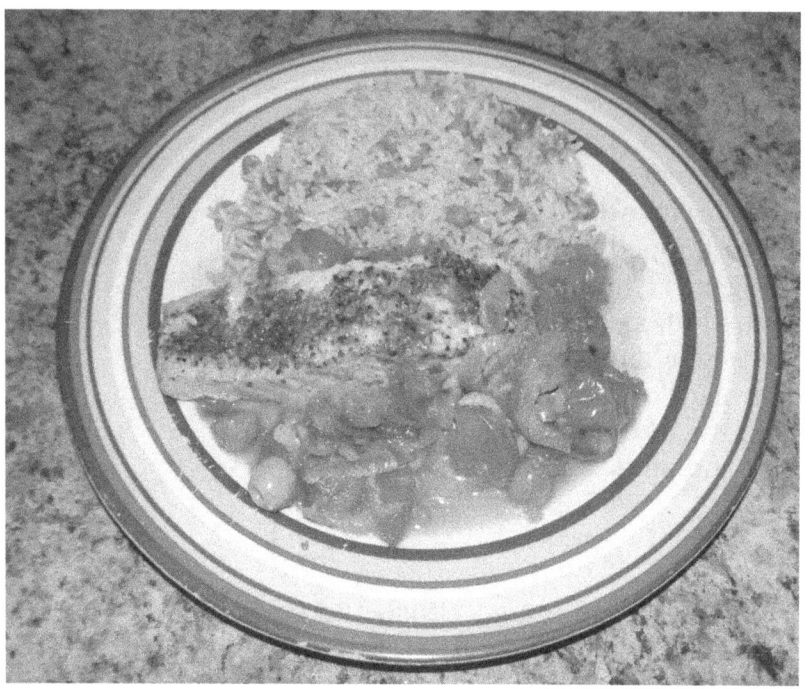

Ingredients

1 tbsp extra virgin olive oil
1 red onion
4 garlic cloves
2 cups cherry tomatoes
1/2 cup chopped olives
1 tsp dried oregano
1 cup orange juice
1 tbsp red wine vinegar
4 salmon fillets
Salt
Freshly ground black pepper
4 spring onions

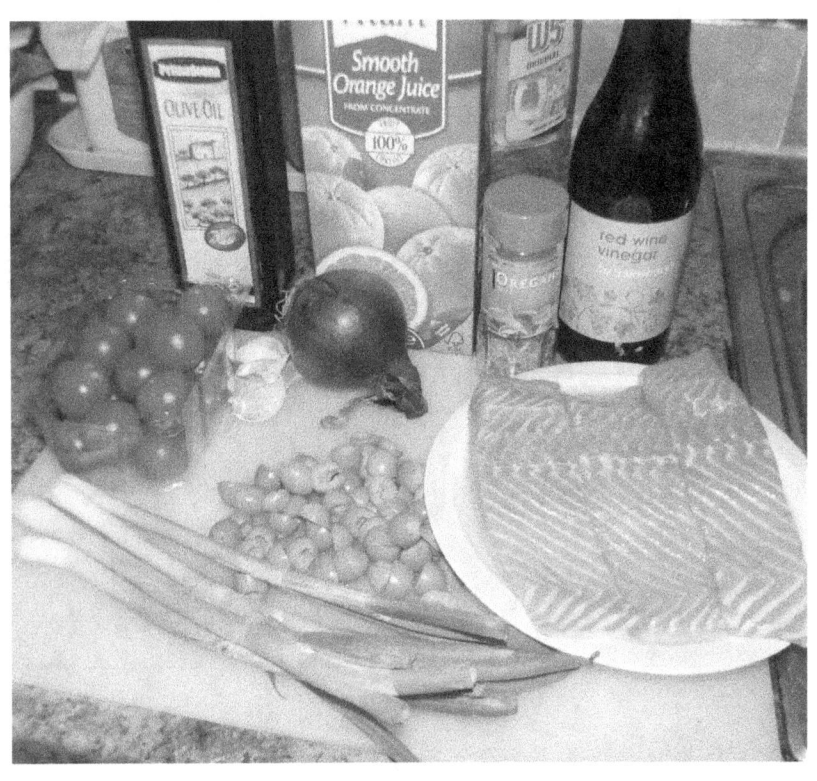

Method

Thinly slice the red onion, spring onions and the garlic.
Cut the tomatoes into halves.

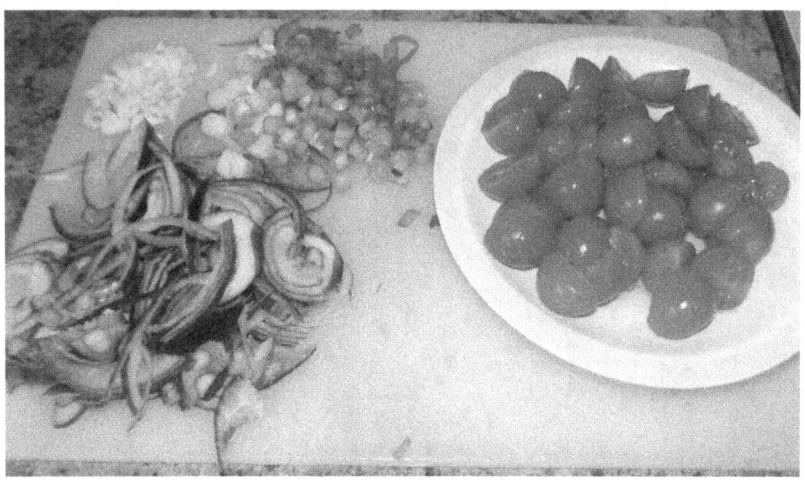

Pat dry the salmon fillets with paper towel and then season the fillets with a little salt and lots of freshly ground black pepper.

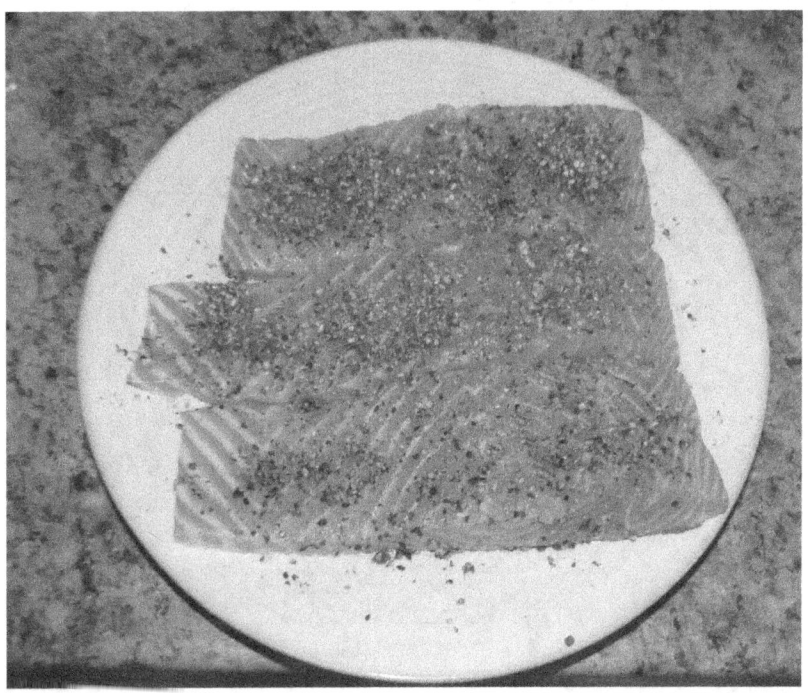

Put the olive oil into a large frying pan and place it on a medium heat. Put in the red onions and garlic and cook gently, while stirring every now and then until they are just lightly browned and nice and soft.

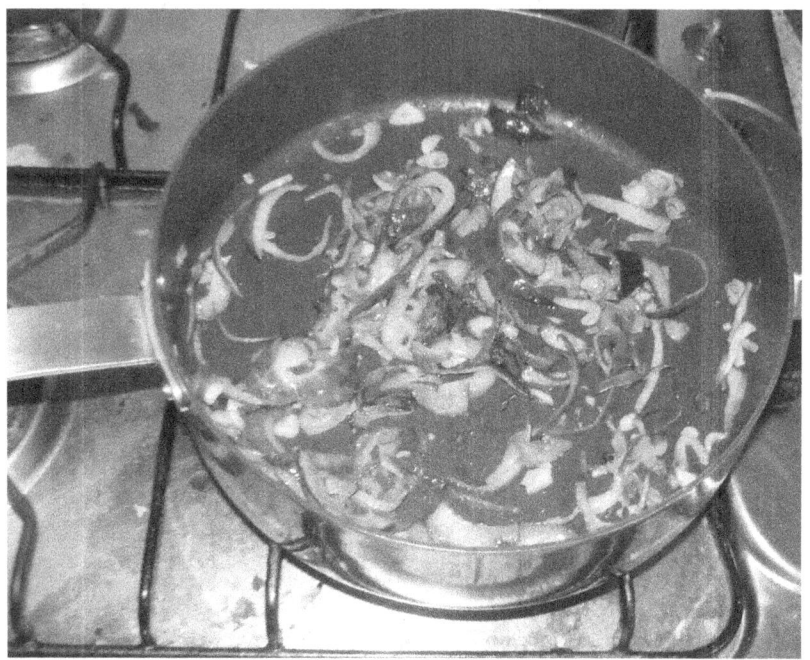

Next stir in the olives, oregano, tomatoes, spring onions, vinegar and orange juice into the pan and continue to cook the mixture for a couple of minutes after it reaches a simmer.

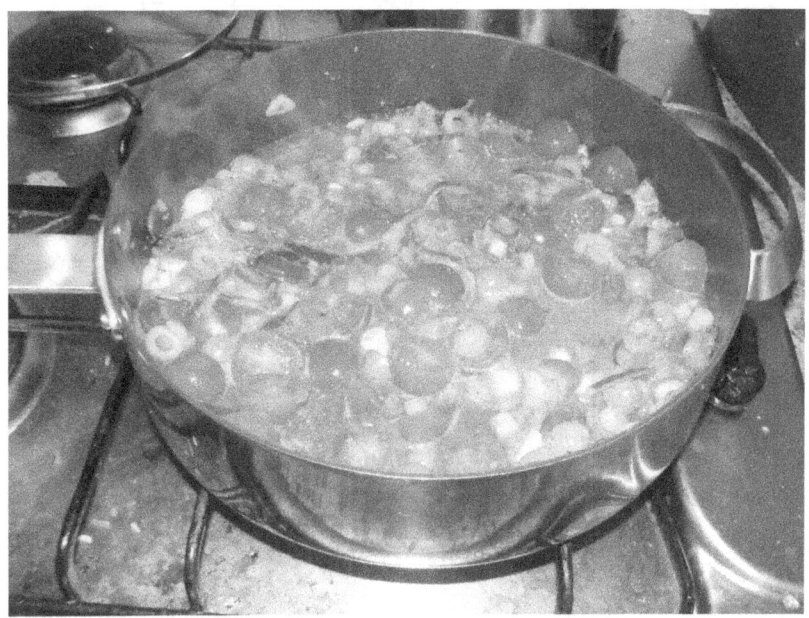

Place the salmon fillets into the tomato mixture in the frying pan and then reduce the heat.

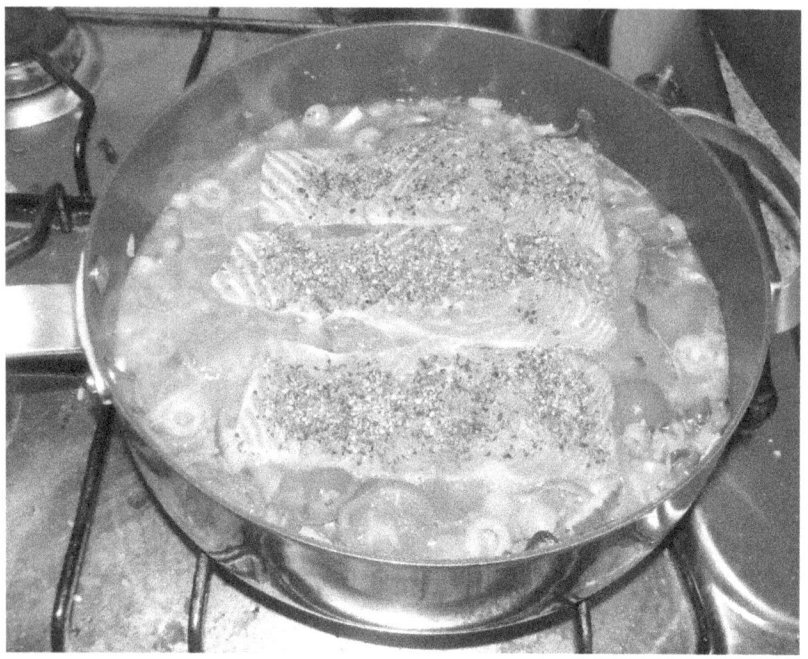

Once the mixture is only just simmering cover the pan with a lid

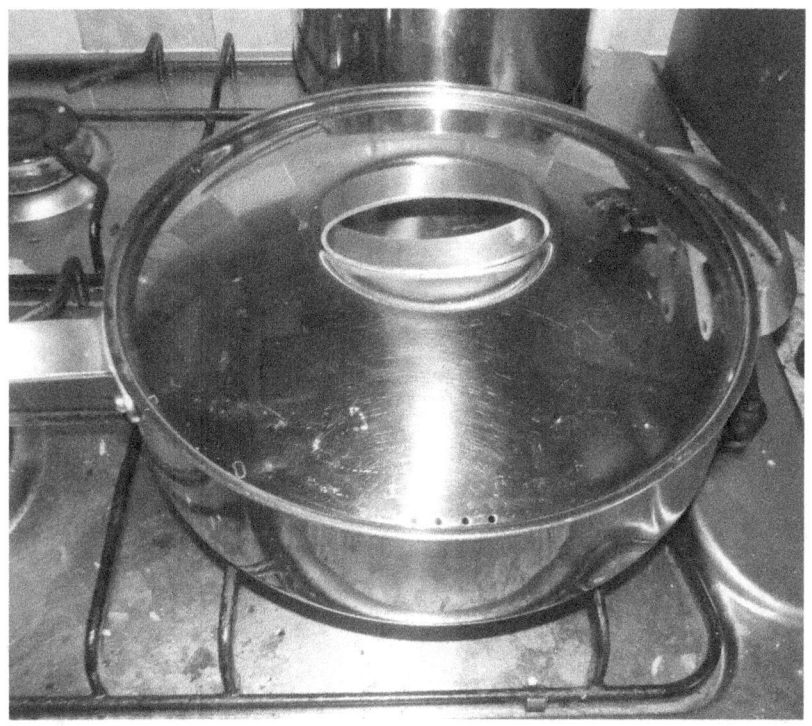

Continue to cook for about fifteen minutes or until the fish is cooked.

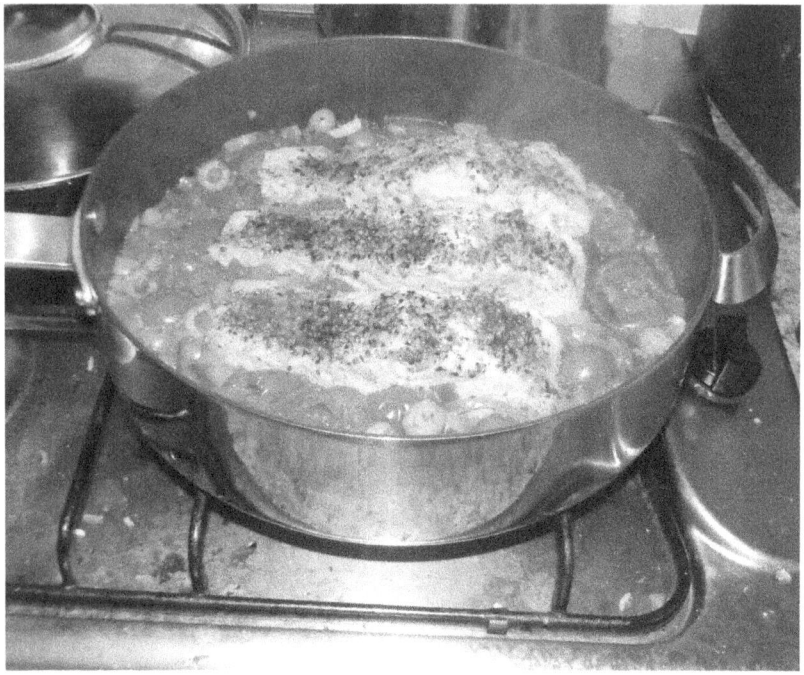

Serve each cooked salmon fillet with a good helping of the tomato sauce from the pan. You can serve this as shown in the plated meal above with whole grain brown rice cooked with peas and fish or vegetable stock.

Green lentils and brown rice

Ingredients

1 cup green lentils
3/4 cup long grain brown rice
3 cups chopped onion
2 tbsp cumin
1 tsp salt
2 tbsp extra virgin olive oil
4 cups water
2 tbsp chopped fresh parsley

Method

Take a large pot or saucepan and add to it the olive oil. Place the pot on a medium to low heat and throw in the onions. Cook the onions until they are nicely browned. Remove about a third of the cooked onions and save for use later in the garnish. Add the rice and the lentils to the remaining onions in the pot and stir them together so that the onions are well combined with the rice and lentils.

Add the water and stir once again. Next add the salt. 1 tsp is suggested but you can add more or less according to your taste. Stir once again and then cook on a medium to low heat for about three quarters of an hour while stirring every now and then. After this time add the cumin, stir and cook for about a further fifteen minutes. Add extra water if it is needed and cook until the lentils are soft.

Once everything is cooked spread it out on a large plate and garnish with the chopped parsley and the browned onions saved from earlier. It is best served with natural yoghurt or salad. It is equally good served hot or cold.

Red lentil soup

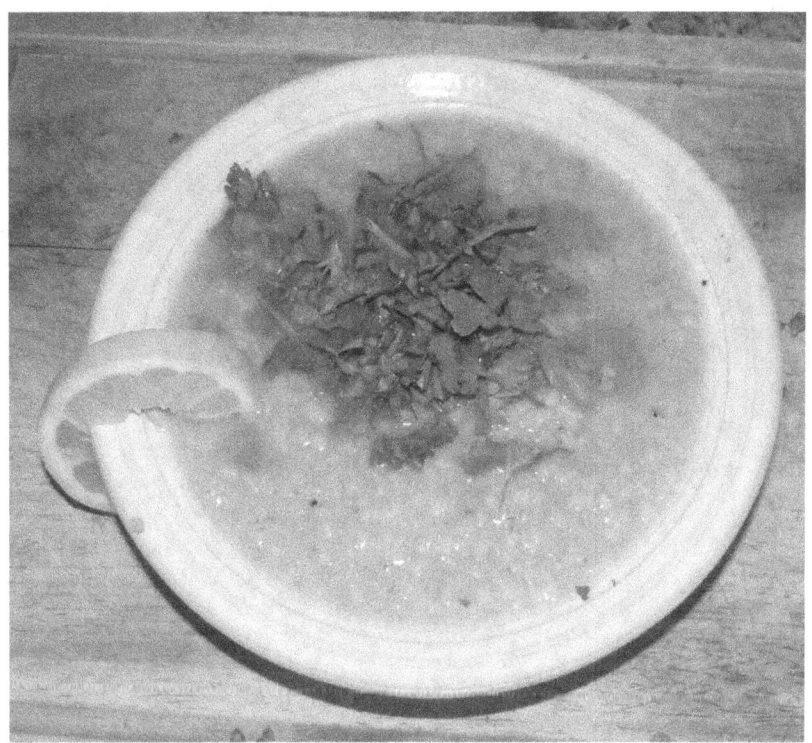

Ingredients

1 cup red lentils
1/2 cup brown rice
1 cup chopped onion
2 chopped garlic cloves
2 cups chopped carrot
1 tsp turmeric
1 tsp cumin
1 tsp ground coriander seed
1/2 tsp salt
1/2 tsp freshly ground black pepper

4 tbsp olive oil
5 cups water
5 cups vegetable stock
1 cup chopped parsley
Lemon juice

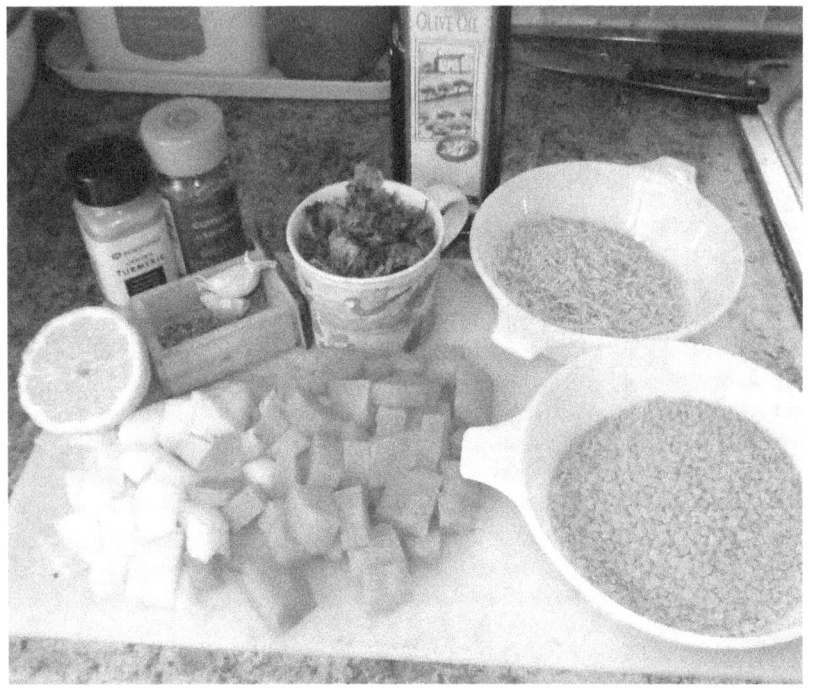

Method

Place the water and the vegetable stock into a large pot. Add the lentils, brown rice and half a teaspoon of salt. Put the pot onto a low heat and cook for about three quarters of an hour.

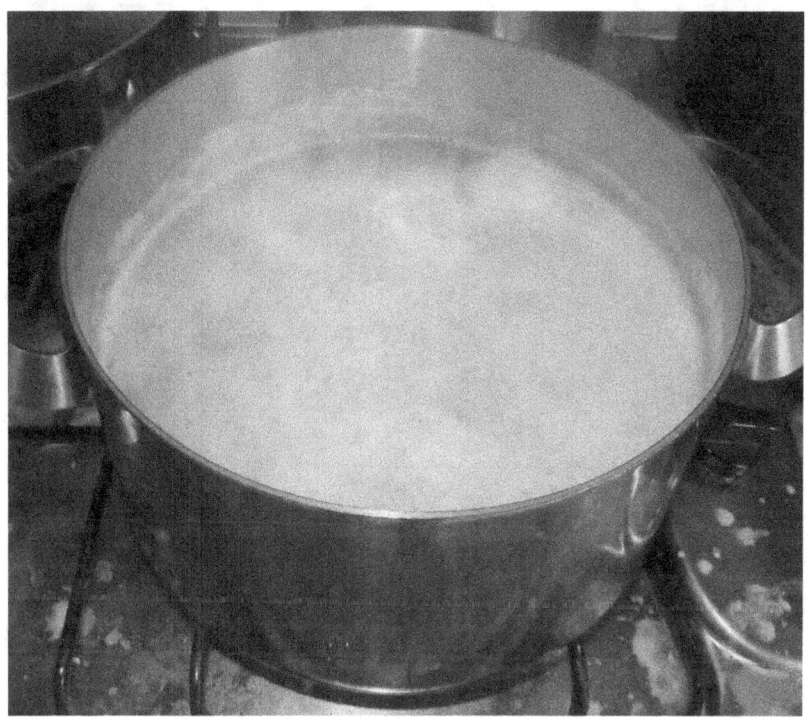

Put the olive oil into a saucepan and place it on a medium heat. Add the chopped onions and garlic and cook them until they are nicely browned.

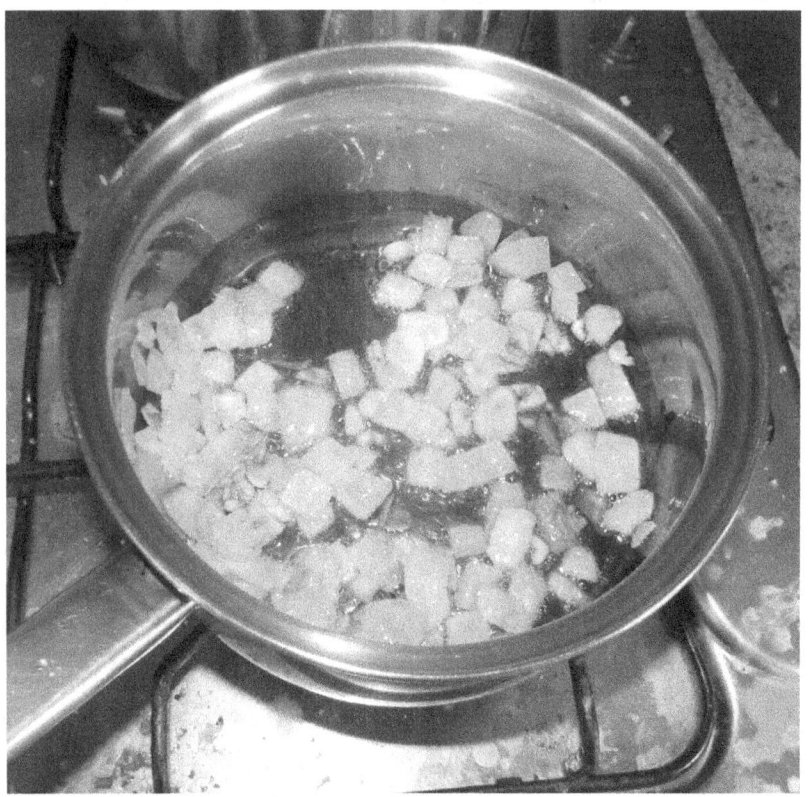

Next add the chopped carrots and continue cooking for a few minutes longer. Once cooked, add the mixture to the soup in the pot.

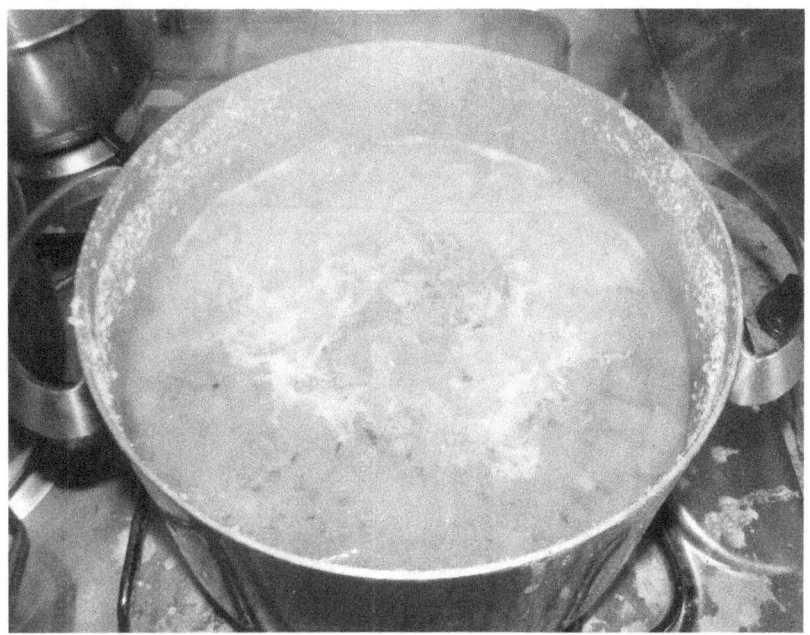

Next add the turmeric, cumin, ground coriander and black pepper and cook for about a further 20 minutes. Adjust the salt seasoning to taste.

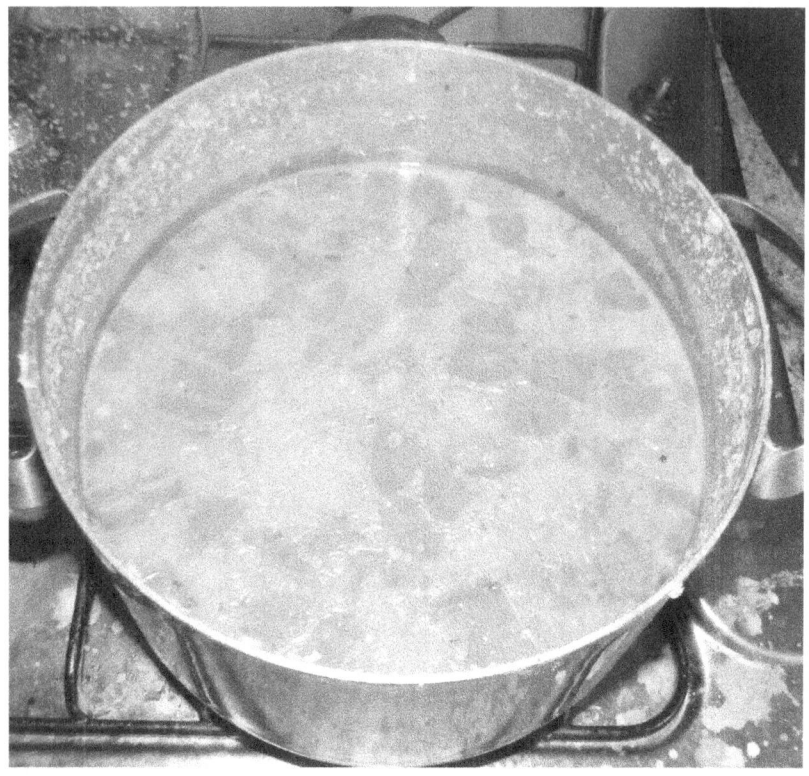

When it is time to serve the soup, garnish each serving with chopped parsley on the top and a little lemon juice. Serve with chunks of whole grain bread.

Further cooking of the soup and general reheating tends to break up the lentils more. Basically cook the soup for as long as it takes to get the consistency that you want.

You can keep the soup for up to five days in the refrigerator. You can add other vegetables such as potatoes or celery to the recipe and you can use a range of chopped herbs for the garnish.

Brown lentils and Bulgur wheat

Ingredients

3 cups chopped onions
2 cups brown lentils
1 cup bulgur wheat
2 tbsp ground cumin
1/2 tsp salt
1 tsp black pepper
1/2 cup olive oil
6 cups water
2 cups coarsely chopped onions

Method

Add the olive oil to a large pot and place it on a medium heat. Add the chopped onions and the salt and cook the onions, while stirring, until they are nicely browned but not burnt.

In a large saucepan put 4 cups of water and heat until it is boiling. Next add the lentils and cook for about fifteen minutes. Pour the water surrounding the lentils into the pot with the onions and then mash the onions. Once they are mashed in the water cook them for about five minutes. Add another two cups of water and then stir in the cooked lentils from the saucepan. Add the cumin, salt and black pepper and cook the mixture while stirring for about a further five minutes. Next add the bulgur wheat and cook while stirring for another five minutes.

For the garnish cook the coarsely chopped onions in a frying pan using a little olive oil. Cook them until they are caramelized. Use a fork to fluff up the lentils in the pot and then serve portions on a plate with some of the caramelized onions on top.

This dish goes well with salad and pita bread and natural yoghurt.

Cannellini beans and sun dried tomatoes

Ingredients

2 cups cooked cannellini beans
1 Portobello mushroom cap
1/4 cup sun dried tomatoes
1 medium garlic clove
2 tbsp minced fresh thyme leaves
2 tbsp extra virgin olive oil
Salt, to taste

Method

Dice the mushroom cap and the sundried tomatoes into small pieces. Mince the garlic clove.

Put the olive oil into a pan and set it on a medium heat. Add the diced mushrooms and cook until they start to brown. Put in the sun dried tomatoes and the minced garlic. Once you can smell the garlic cooking add the beans to the pan and stir them in so that they become coated with the oil mixture. Next put in the thyme and cook for just a little longer. Add salt to taste and then serve while still hot.

White bean and avocado salad

Ingredients

2 avocados
1/2 pint cherry tomatoes
1 chopped garlic clove
1/2 large red onion
1/2 cup coriander
1/2 red bell pepper
1/2 green bell pepper
1 cup cooked cannellini beans
1/4 cup olive oil
Juice of 1 lime
Salt
Freshly ground black pepper

Method

Peel the avocados and then cut them into chunks. Cut the cherry tomatoes into halves. Mince the red onion. Finely chop the coriander. Remove the seeds from the bell peppers and finely chop them.

Mix the avocados, cherry tomatoes, red onion, garlic, coriander, red pepper, green pepper, cannellini beans together in a large bowl. Drizzle the olive oil in a swirl pattern over the contents of the bowl and add the lime juice. Season the mixture to taste with salt and freshly ground black pepper and then stir to blend everything together. Serve the salad at room temperature. This is a perfect dish for a light lunch in the middle of summer.

Judias Verdes with potato and peppers

This recipe is based on the classic Spanish dish using green beans. In my opinion runner beans are the best choice although you can do a fair job with French beans too.

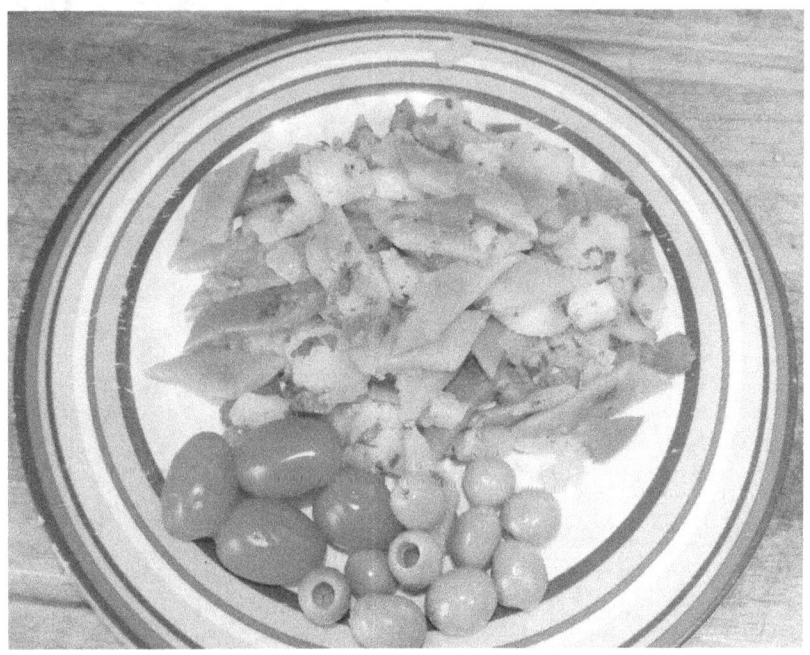

Ingredients

250g green beans (Runner or French)
2 medium potatoes
1 onion
1/2 green pepper
1/2 red pepper
1 or 2 garlic cloves
2 tbsp extra virgin olive oil

1 chilli (optional)
Freshly ground black pepper
Small handful of Fresh parsley

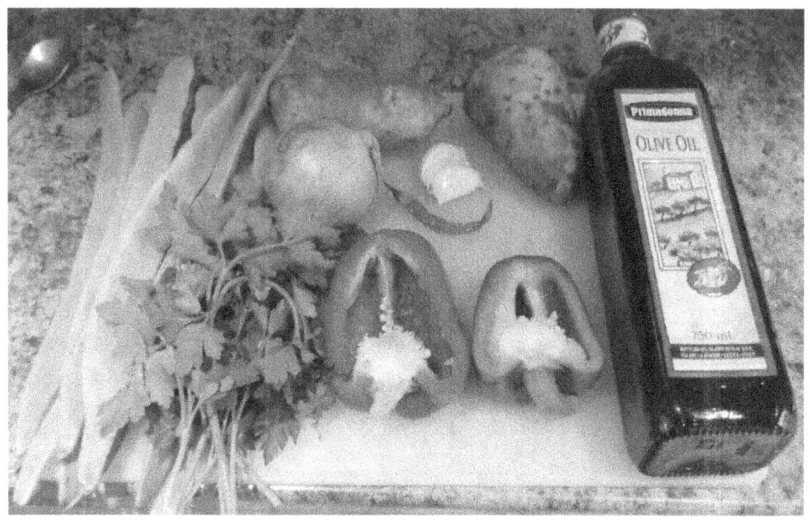

Method

Top and tail the runner beans and then cut them diagonally to give pleasing shapes.

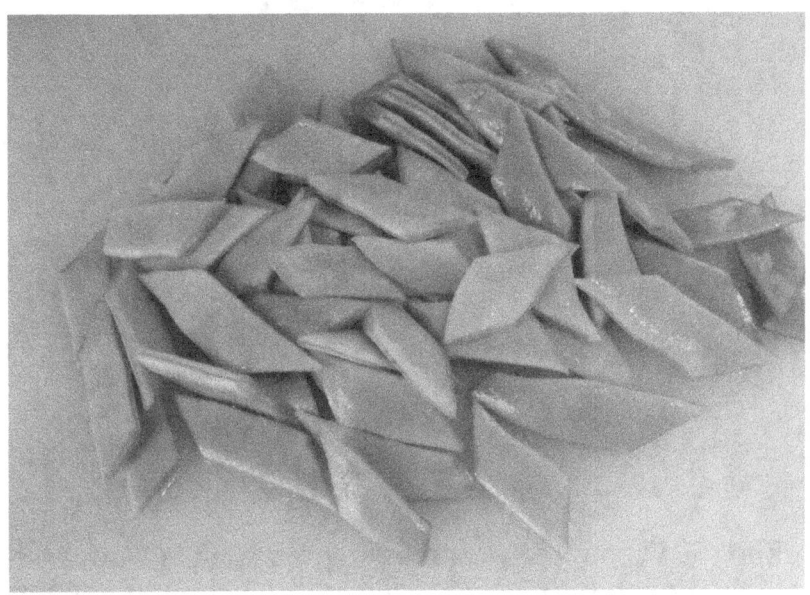

Peel and dice the potatoes into cubes of about 1cm in size.

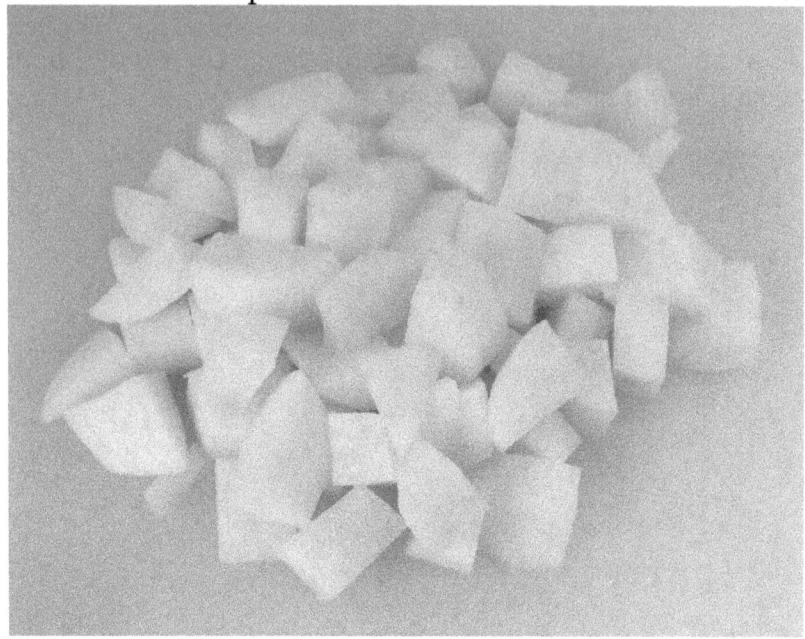

Chop the Onion, red pepper and green pepper into small pieces. Roughly chop the garlic and the chilli, if you are including it.

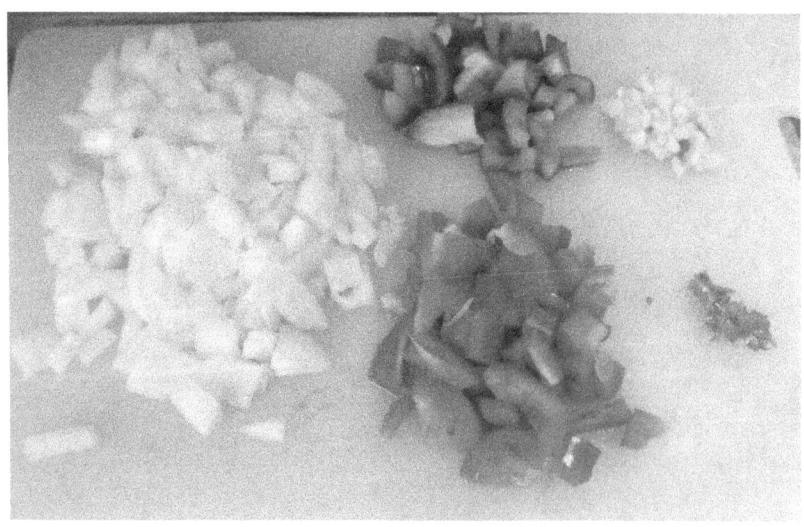

Cook the diced potatoes for about 10 minutes so that they are partly boiled. The potato cubes should still be firm. Drain the water from the part cooked potatoes.

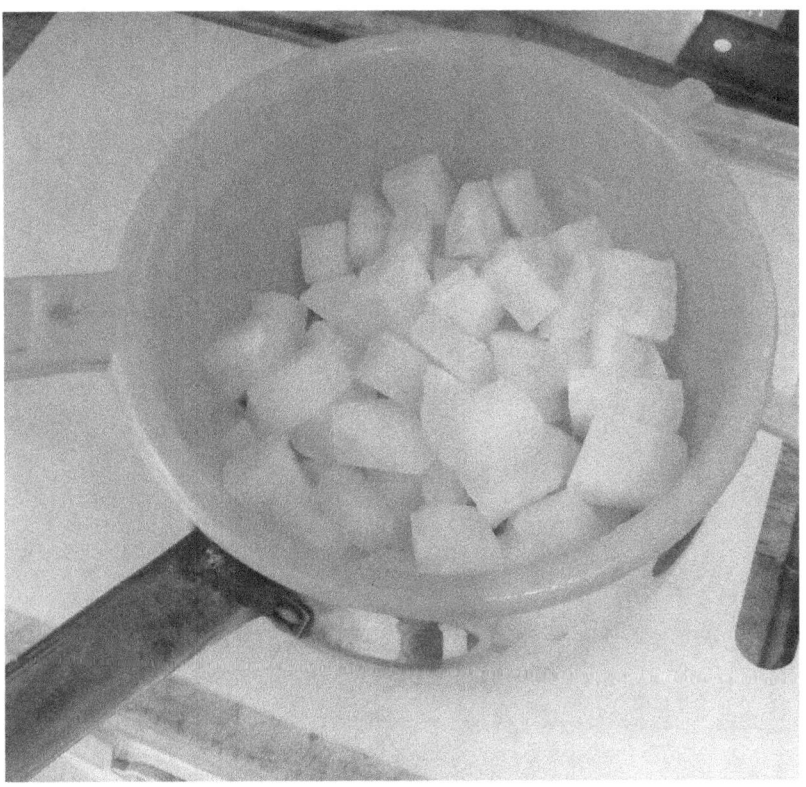

Boil the green beans for about 15 minutes. They should be tender but not over cooked.

While the beans are cooking put the olive oil into a large deep frying pan and set on a medium to low heat. Put the chopped onion and chilli into the pan and gently cook until the onions become transparent and soft.

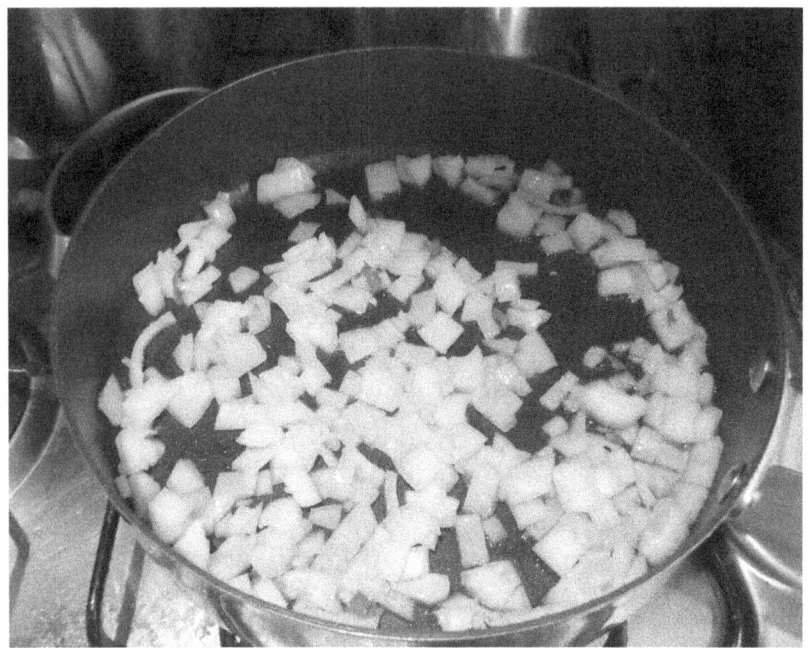

Add the part cooked potato to the pan and continue cooking for about another 5 minutes.

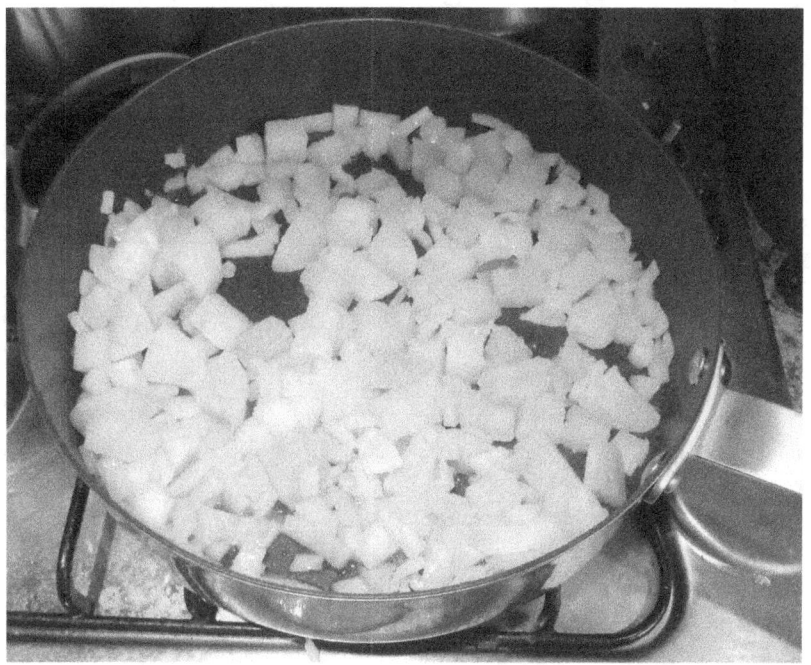

Add the green and red pepper together with the garlic to the pan and cook for a couple of further minutes. The potato should now be fully cooked but still firm.

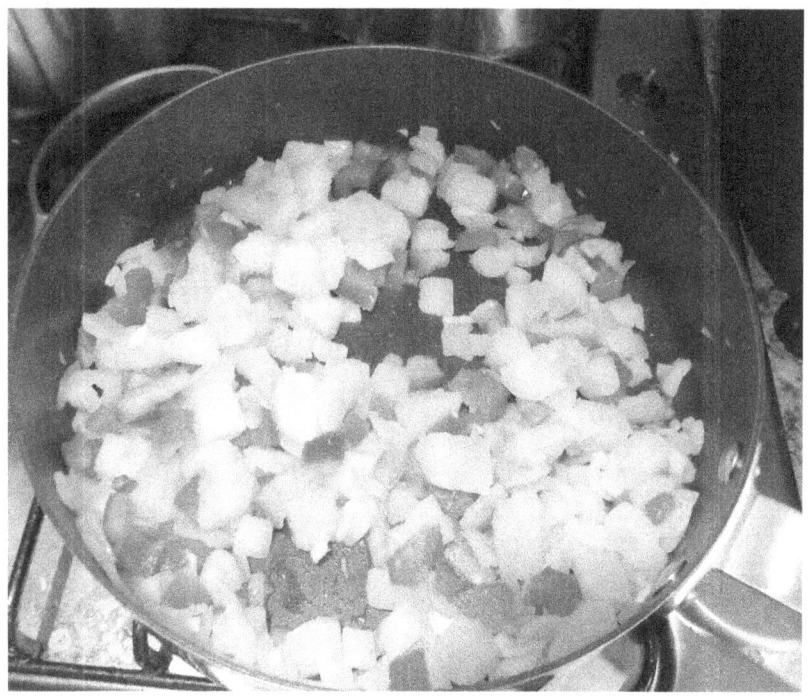

Roughly chop the parsley and add it to the pan.

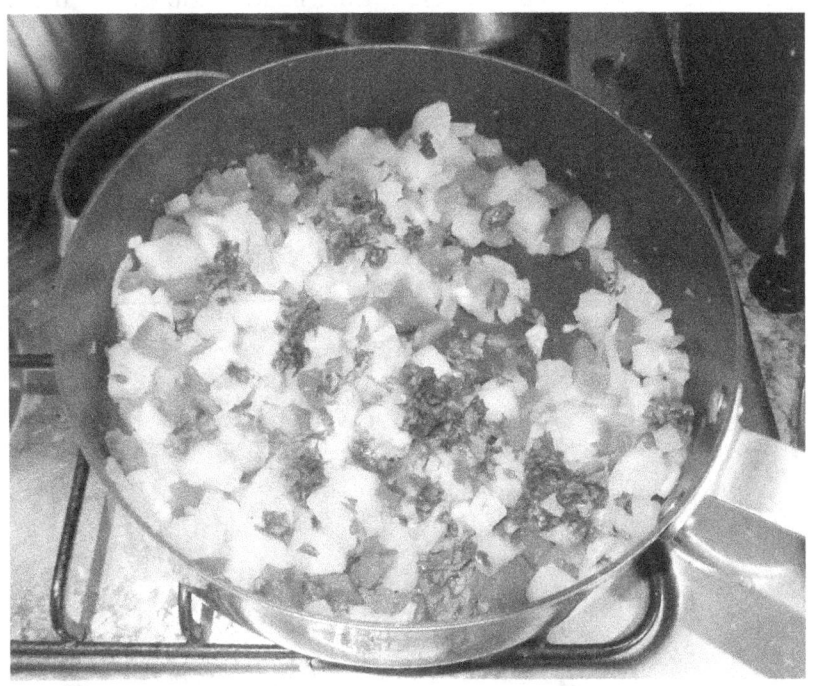

Add the cooked chopped beans to the pan and mix all of the ingredients together. Continue cooking until everything is heated through.

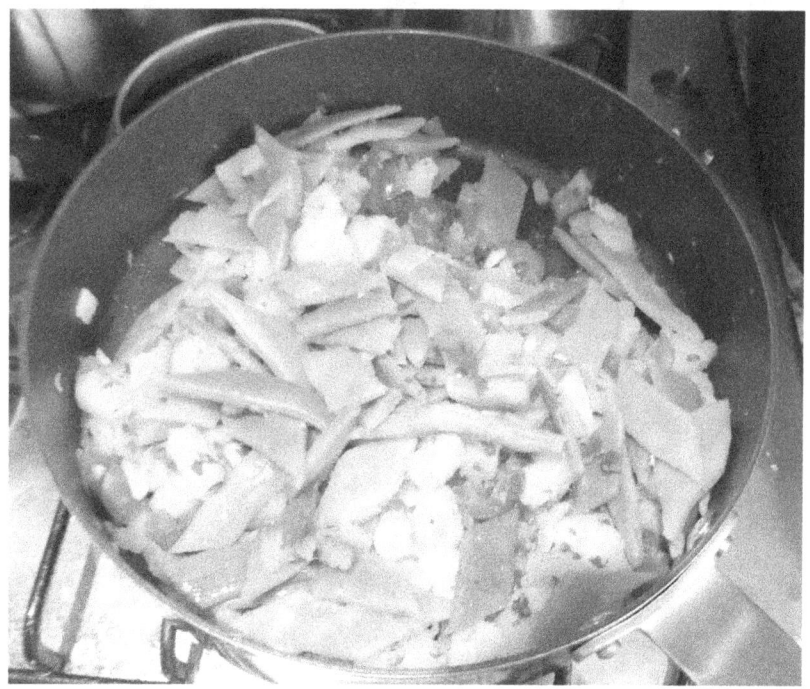

Season to taste with freshly ground black pepper and salt if needed. Serve the Judias Verdes while hot with pitted olives and cherry or cherry plum tomatoes.

You can experiment by adding other ingredients such as chopped mushrooms or chopped cooked carrot for variation. You can also add other fresh herbs that maybe available instead of or as well as the parsley.

Prawn fried rice

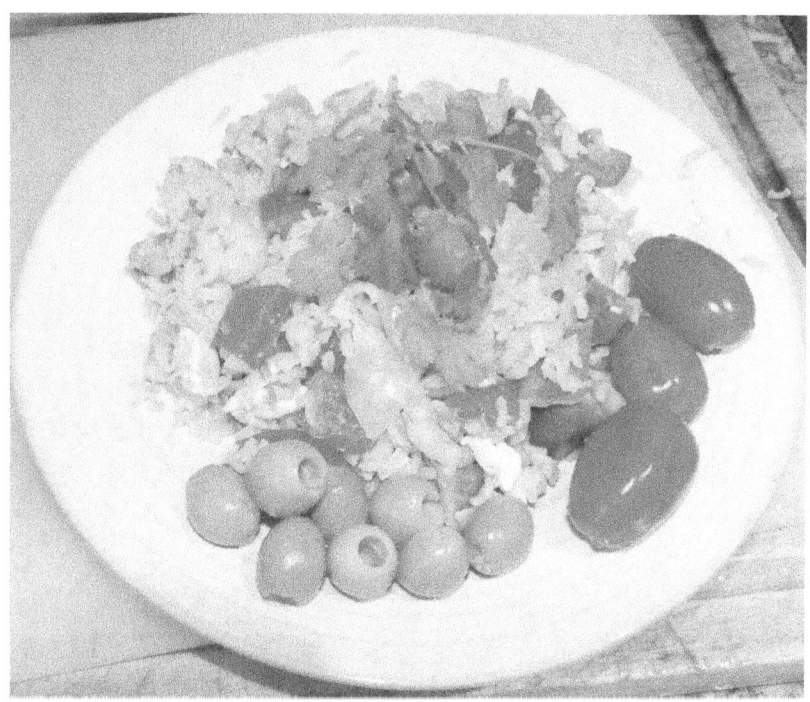

Ingredients

300g cooked peeled prawns
400g brown long grain rice
1 onion
1/2 green pepper
1/2 red pepper
50g sun dried tomatoes
2 eggs
Handful mange tout
Bunch coriander
2-3 garlic cloves
1 chilli (fresh or dried)

1 inch ginger stem
2 tbsp extra virgin olive oil + more for frying eggs
Freshly ground black pepper
Salt

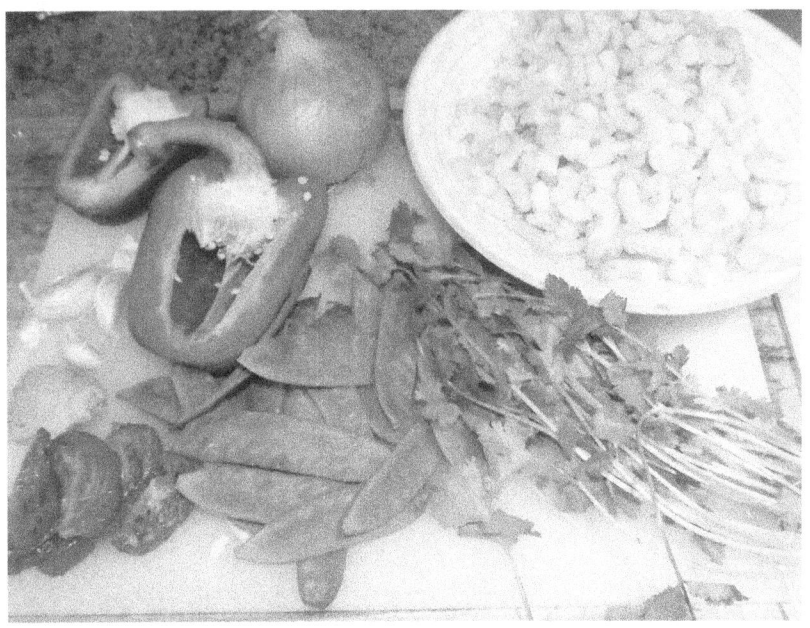

Method

Cook the brown rice in the usual way that you use. Cook until the grains are tender but still a little firm.

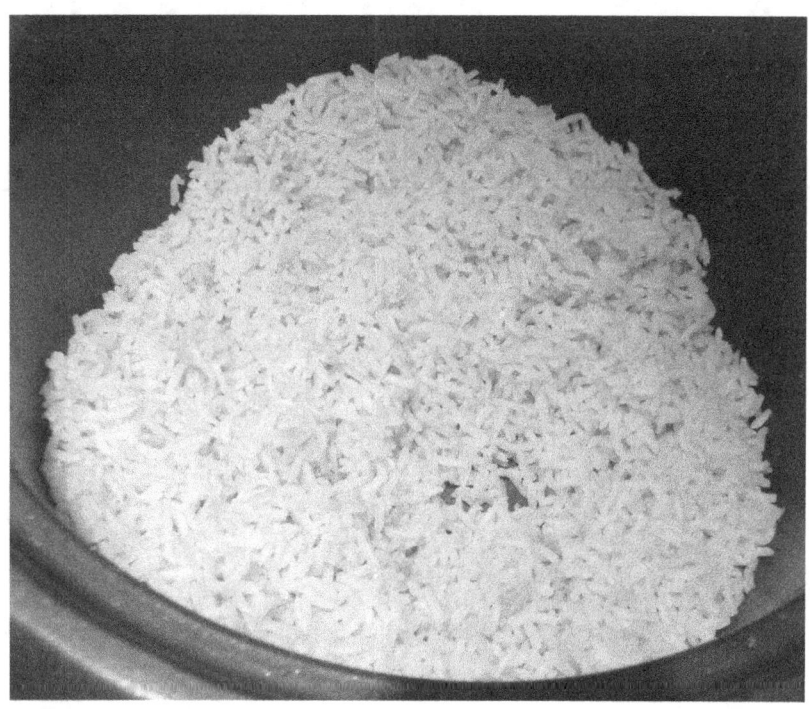

While the rice is cooking chop the onion, ginger and chilli.

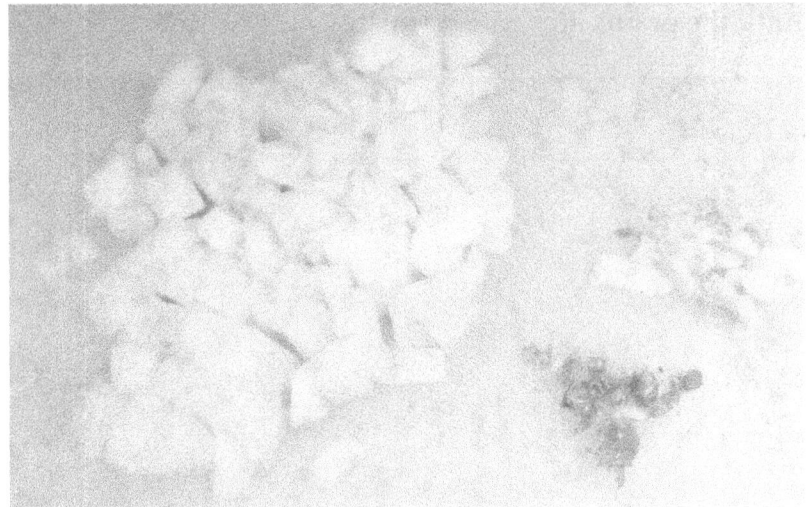

Put the 2 tbsp olive oil into a large deep frying pan and put onto a medium to low heat. Add the chopped, onion, ginger and chilli. Cook gently until the onions are soft and transparent.

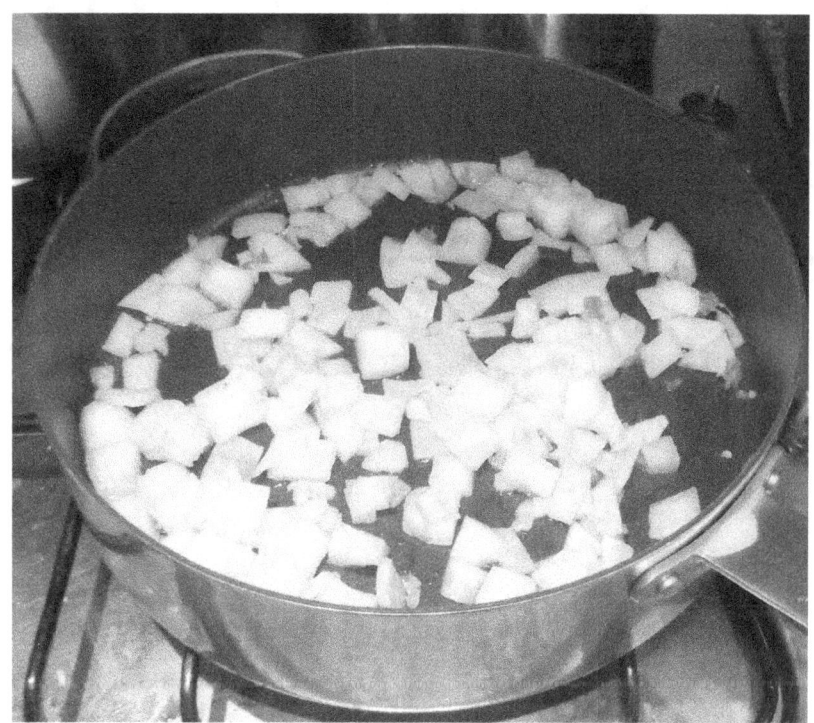

While the onions are cooking chop the red pepper, green pepper and garlic cloves. Cut the mange tout and sundried tomatoes into suitable sizes using scissors or a sharp knife.

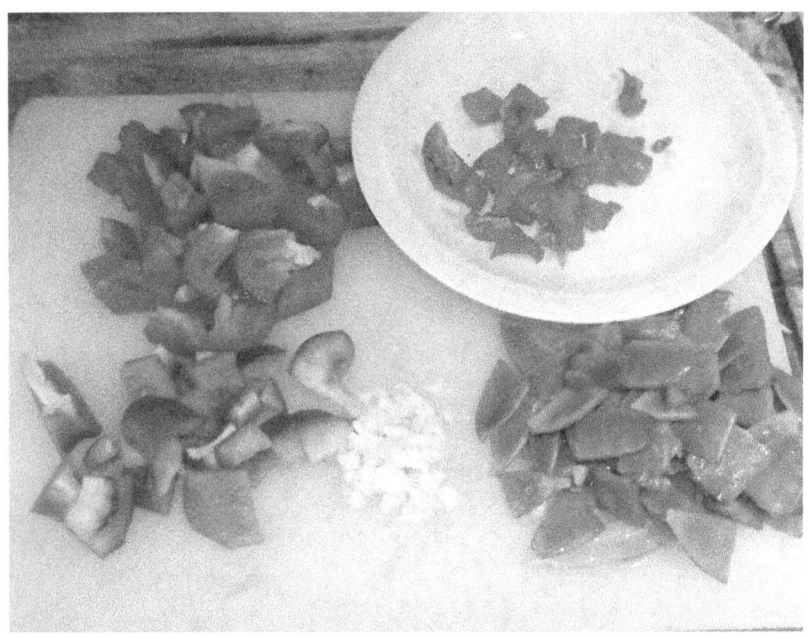

Add the red pepper, green pepper, mange tout and garlic to the pan and continue cooking for about another 5 minutes.

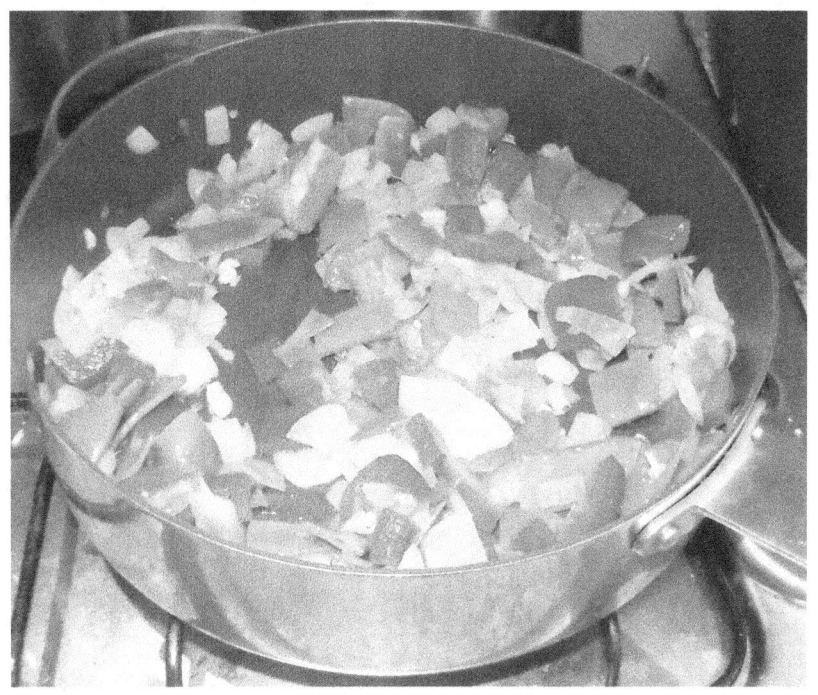

Add the prawns and sun dried tomatoes to the pan and continue to cook gently. The aim is to only heat the prawns through as they are already cooked. Do not cook fiercely as the prawns will shrink in size. If the prawns you use are of the frozen variety you may need to heat the pan for longer to thaw them out first.

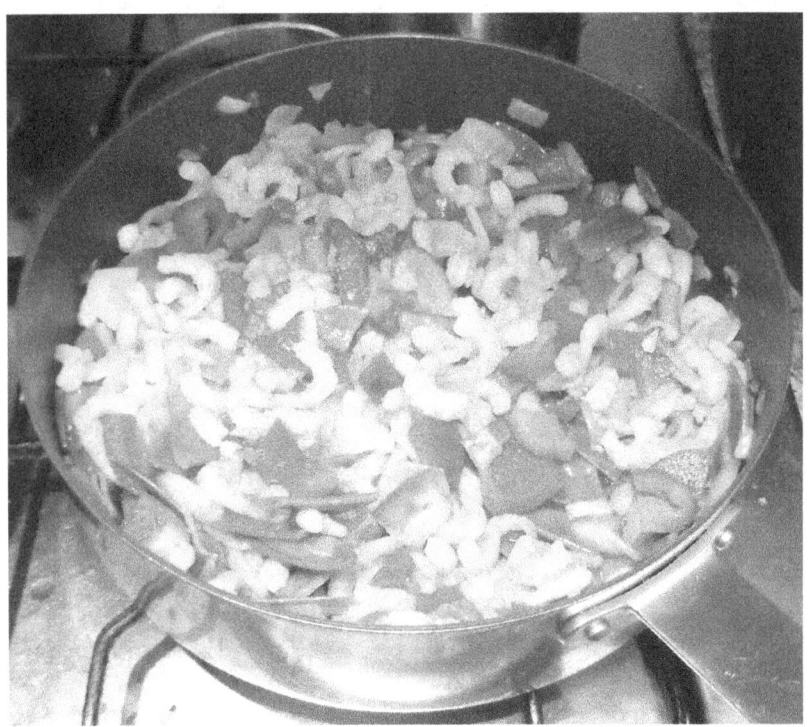

While the prawns are heating crack 2 eggs into another smaller frying pan with a little olive oil. Rupture the yolks and fry the eggs turning them to cook both sides.

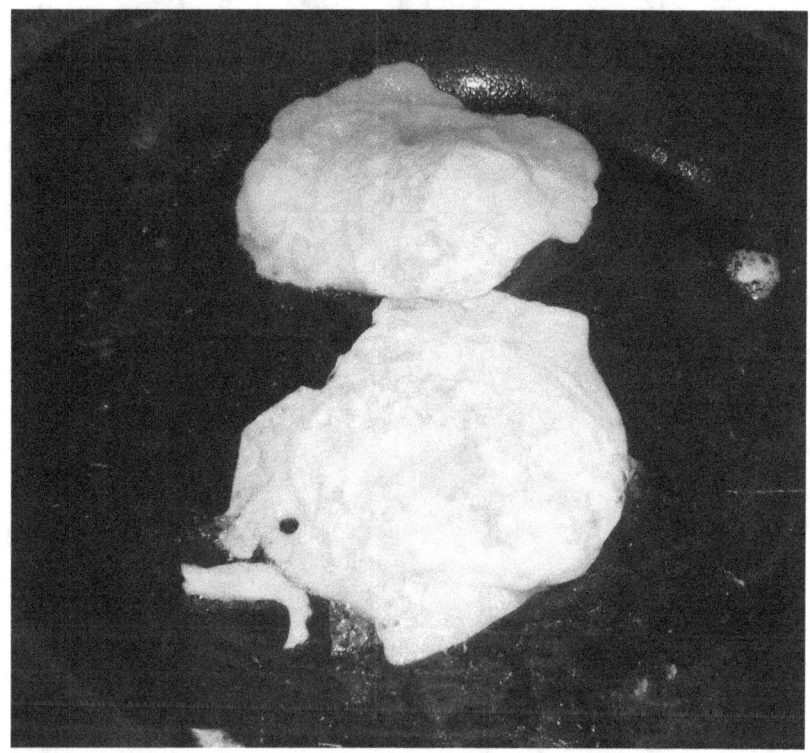

Use 2 wooden spatulas to break up the fried eggs into small pieces.

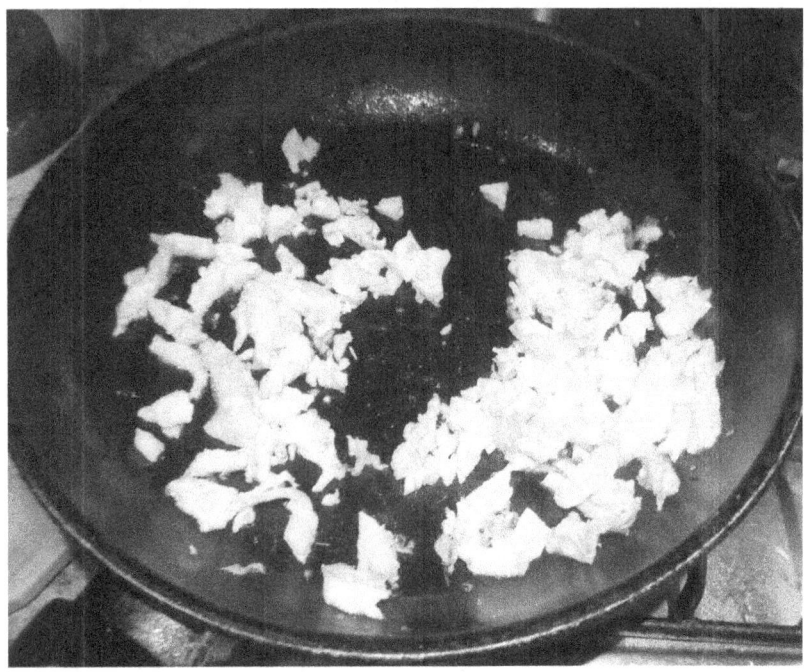

Chop the coriander and add it together with the pieces of fried egg to the prawn mixture in the other pan and stir to combine.

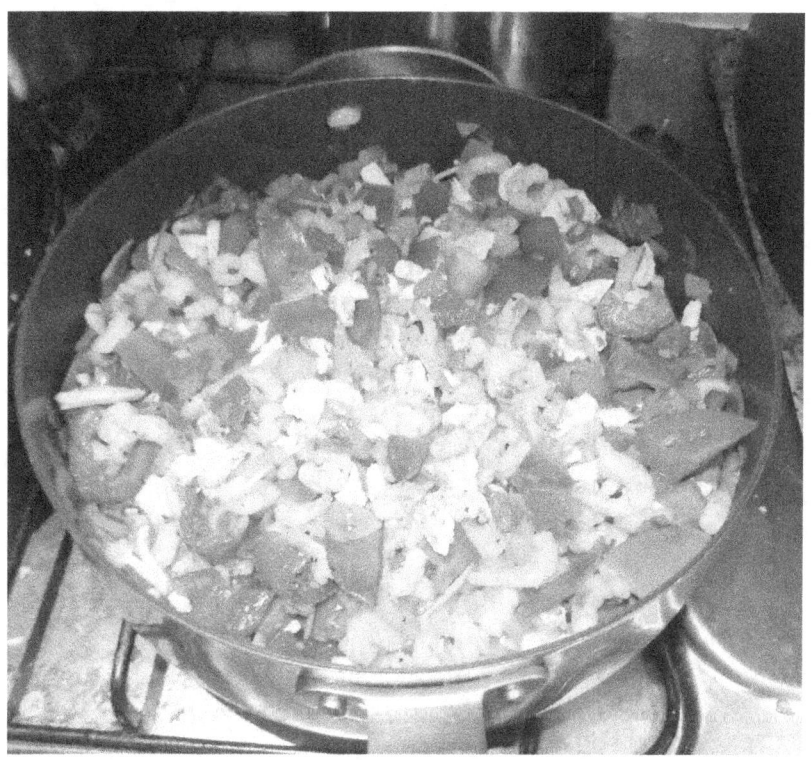

Add the cooked brown rice to the pan and toss the prawn mixture with the wooden spatulas to combine it with the rice.

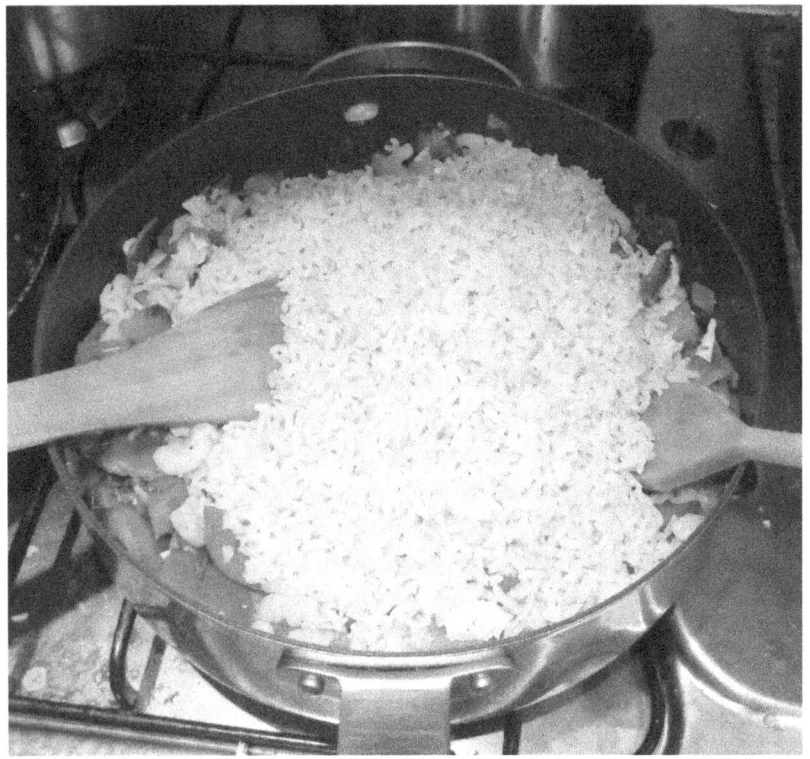

Once everything is fully combined adjust the seasoning with freshly ground black pepper and salt if needed. The dish is now ready to serve.

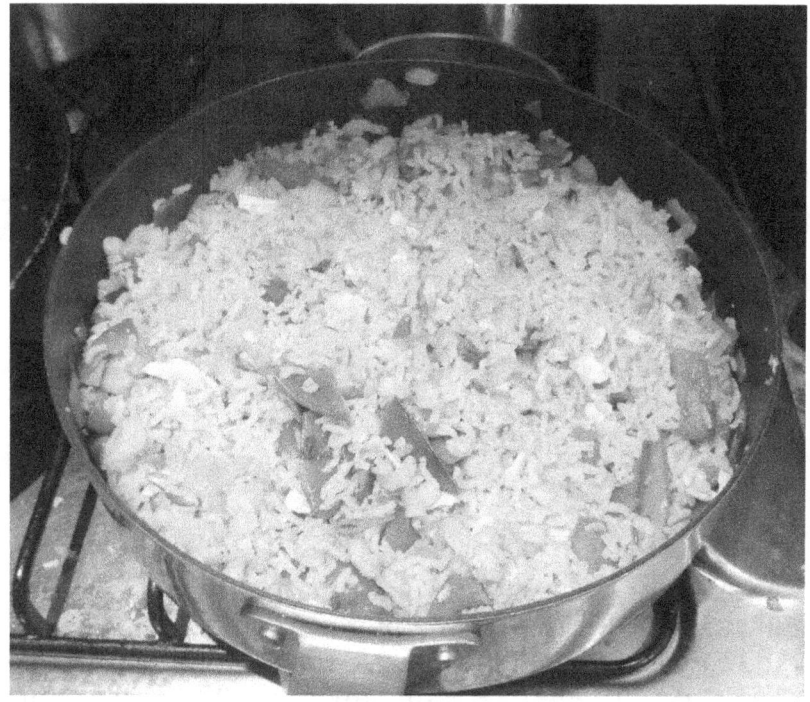

Garnish on plates with sprigs of coriander, olives and cherry or mini plum tomatoes. You can add lemon juice to complement the prawns and or soy sauce to give a more Chinese style to the dish.

Tomato risotto with brown rice

Ingredients

50 ml extra virgin olive oil
3/4 cup short grain brown rice
50 ml white wine
2 cups vegetable stock
1 tsp salt
1/2 tsp coarsely ground pepper
3 cups baby spinach leaves
1 tbsp roughly chopped sun dried tomatoes
1 tbsp roughly chopped olives
1 tbsp grated Parmesan cheese

Method

Put the olive oil into a large pan and heat it on a low heat. Put the brown rice into the pan and stir it so that all of the brown rice is covered by the olive oil. Add the white wine and continue to stir the mixture until the wine has evaporated.

Season with the salt and pepper and then add the vegetable stock. Increase the heat and continue to stir until the mixture boils. Cover the pan with a lid and then lower the heat to a simmer. Simmer the mixture for about 10 minutes and then turn off the heat. Don't remove the pan lid. And leave the risotto to stand for a further 10 minutes. After this time stir in the spinach followed by the sun dried tomatoes, chopped olives and the Parmesan cheese. Serve the risotto straight away while it is still nice and hot.

Tomato risotto with whole barley grain

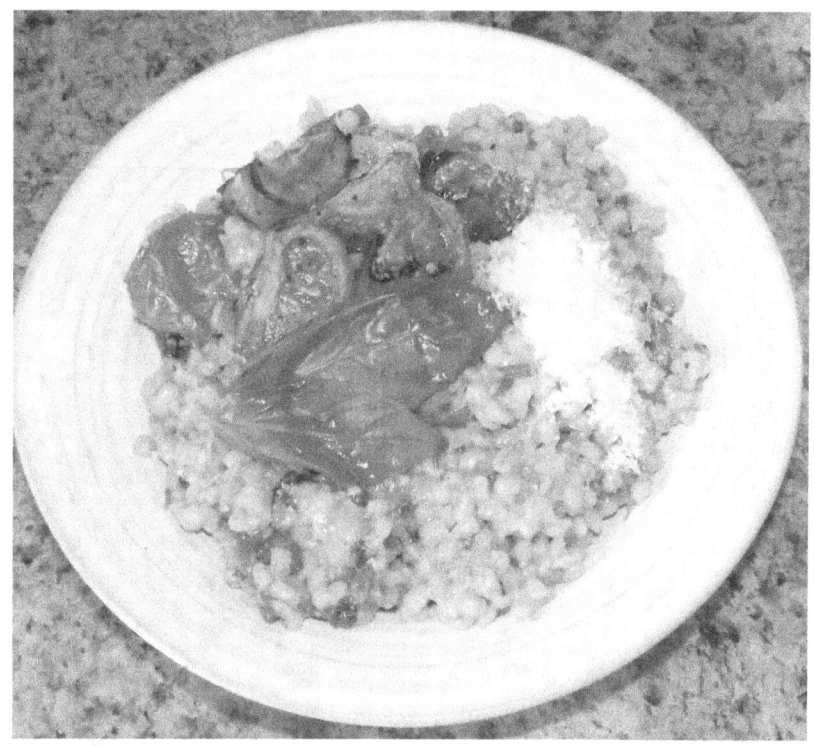

Ingredients

10 large plum tomatoes
2 tablespoons extra virgin olive oil
1 tsp salt
1/2 tsp freshly ground black pepper
4 cups vegetable stock
3 cups water
2 shallots
1/4 cup dry white wine (Optional)
2 cups pearl barley
3 tbsp chopped fresh basil

3 tbsp chopped fresh parsley
1 1/2 tbsp chopped fresh thyme
1/2 cup grated Parmesan cheese

Garnish

Whole fresh basil leaves.
Grated Parmesan cheese

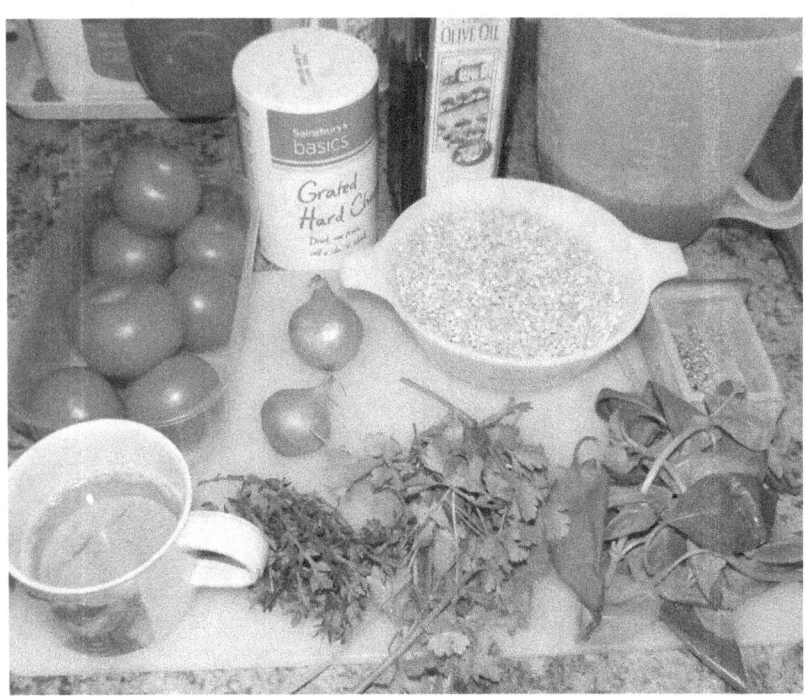

Method

Chop the tomatoes so that each is made up of four wedge shapes. Chop the shallots. Preheat the oven, setting it to 230C.

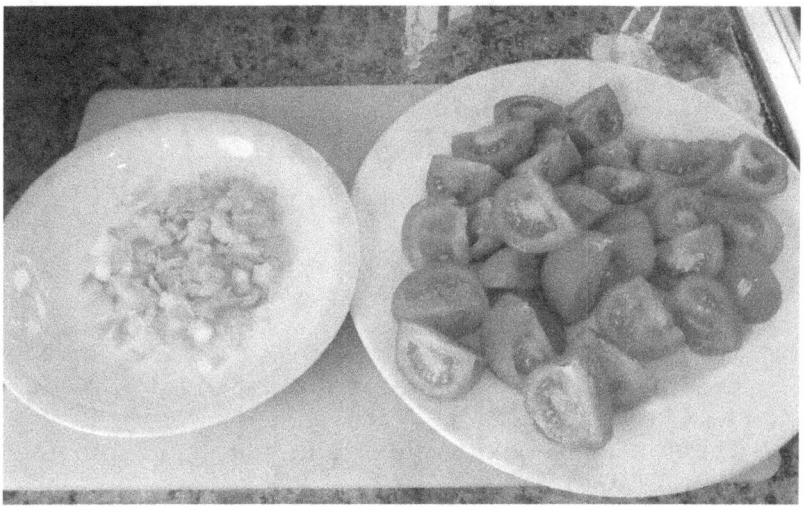

Put the chopped tomatoes in a bowl and then add 1 tbsp of the olive oil. Add a quarter tsp each of salt and black pepper. Gently toss the tomatoes to cover them with the oil mixture.

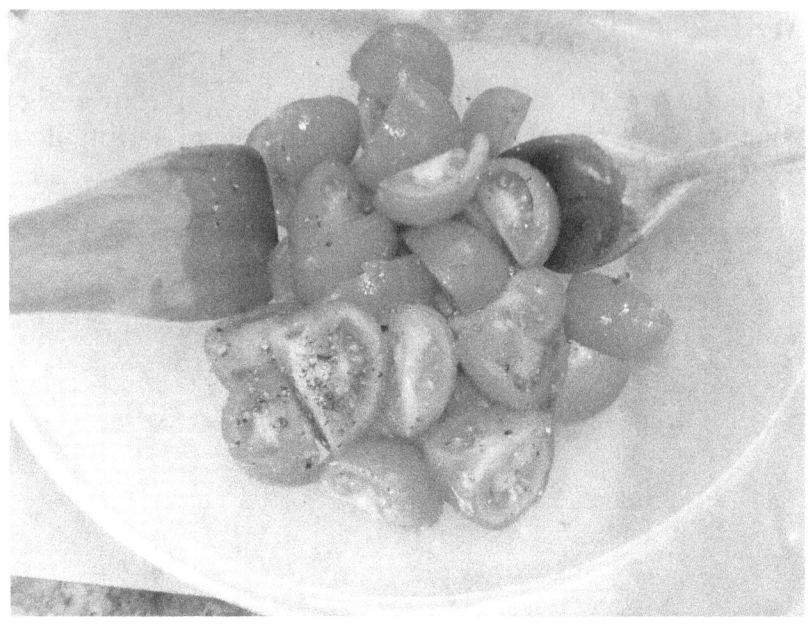

Take a non stick baking sheet and place the tomatoes individually on it.

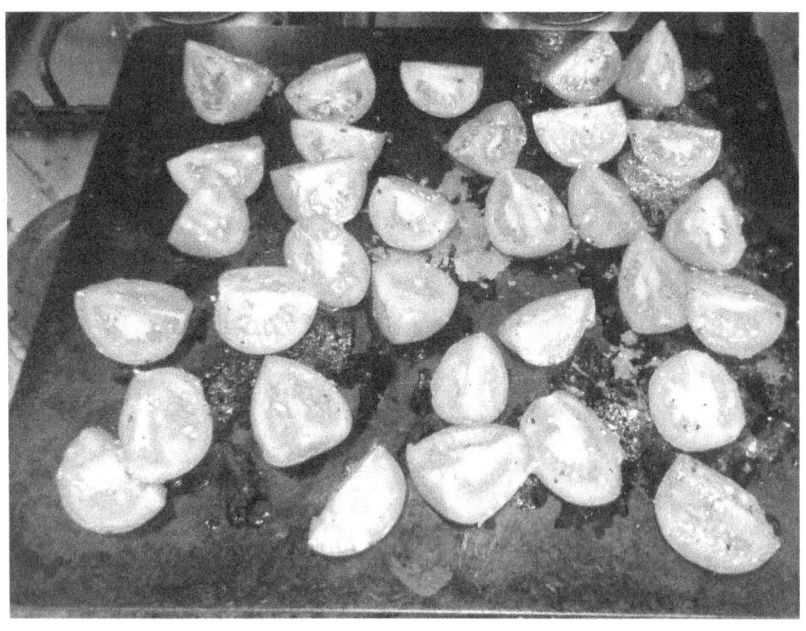

Bake the tomatoes in the oven until they are soft and browned. Keep about 12 of the cooked tomato wedges for the garnish.

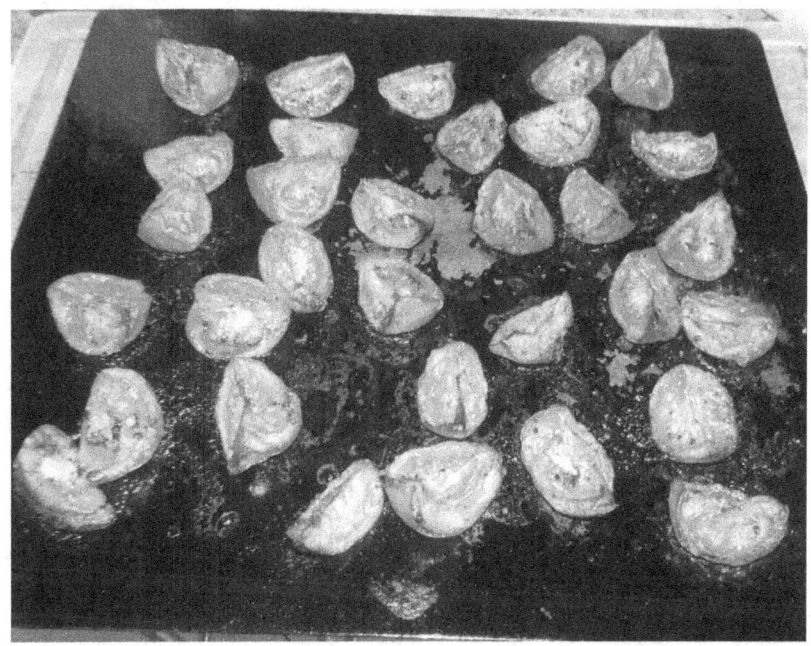

Put the vegetable stock and water into a pan on a high heat and cook until boiling. Reduce the heat so that the stock continues to simmer.

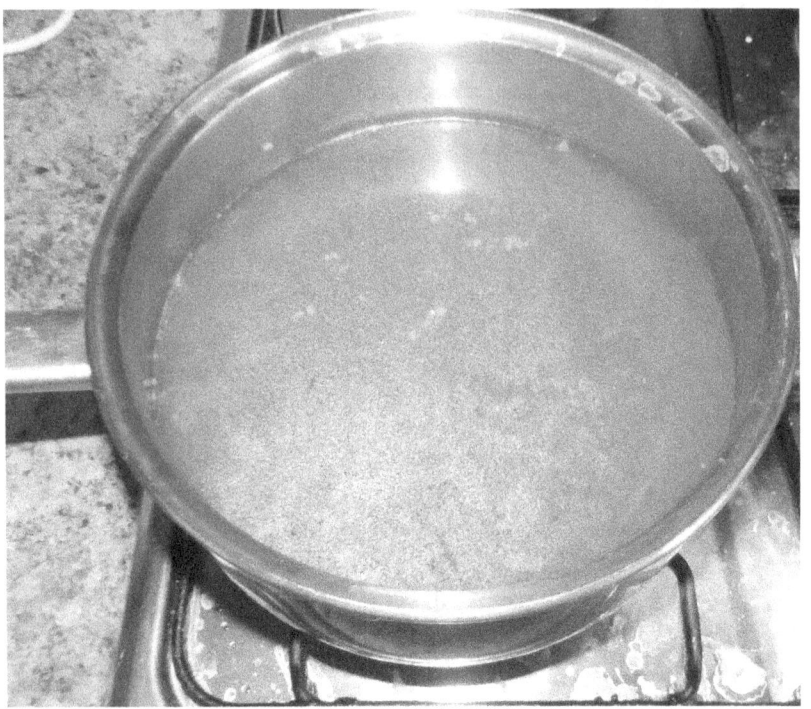

In another pan gently fry the chopped shallots in 1 tbsp of olive oil until they are soft.

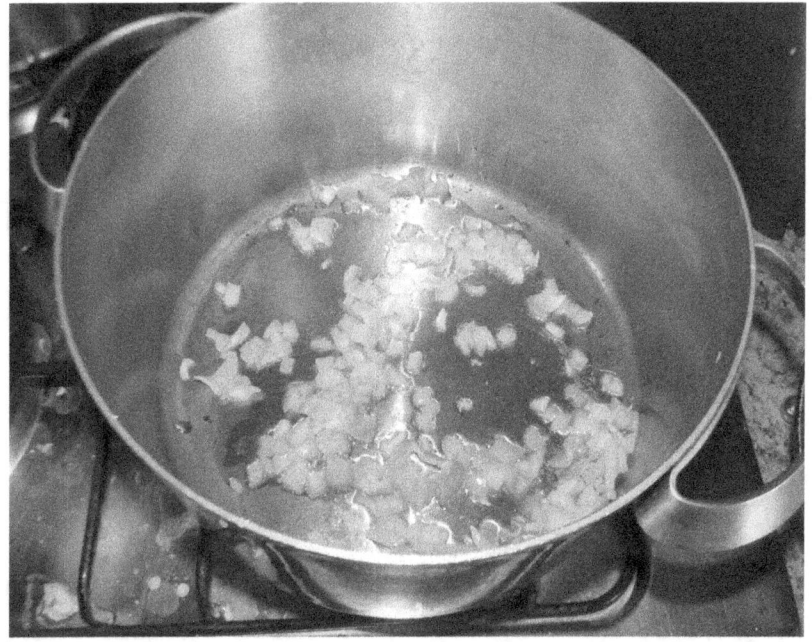

Add the white wine and continue heating until most of it has evaporated.

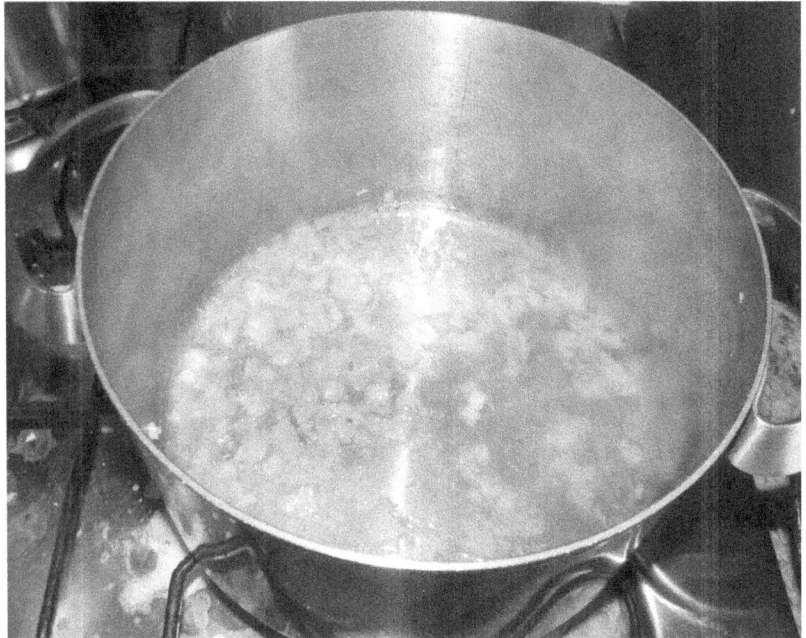

Add the barley and cook for another minute.

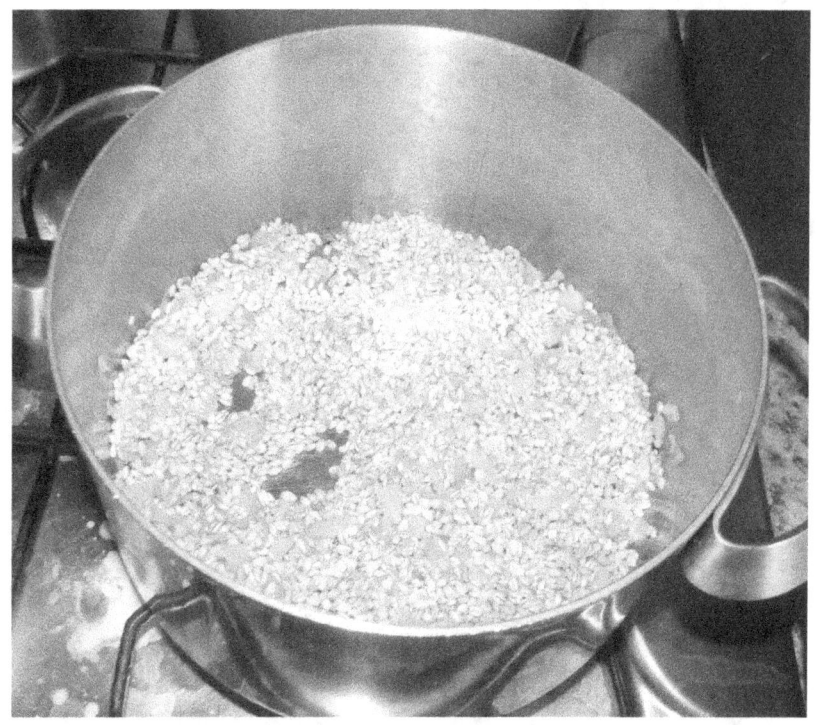

Add half a cup of the chicken stock mixture and cook until the barley absorbs the liquid.

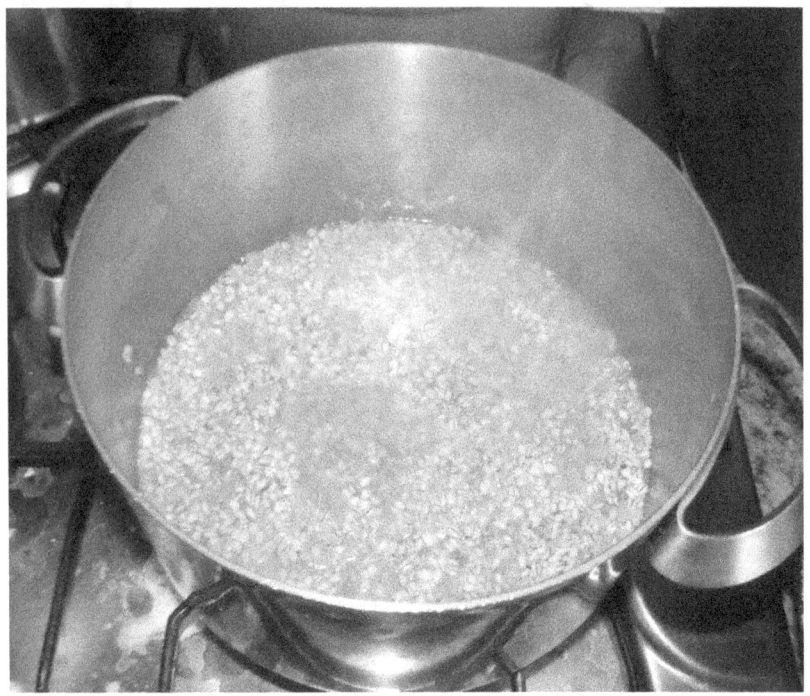

Carry on adding the stock mixture in the same way, half a cup at a time followed by cooking, until the barley is nice and tender and swollen.

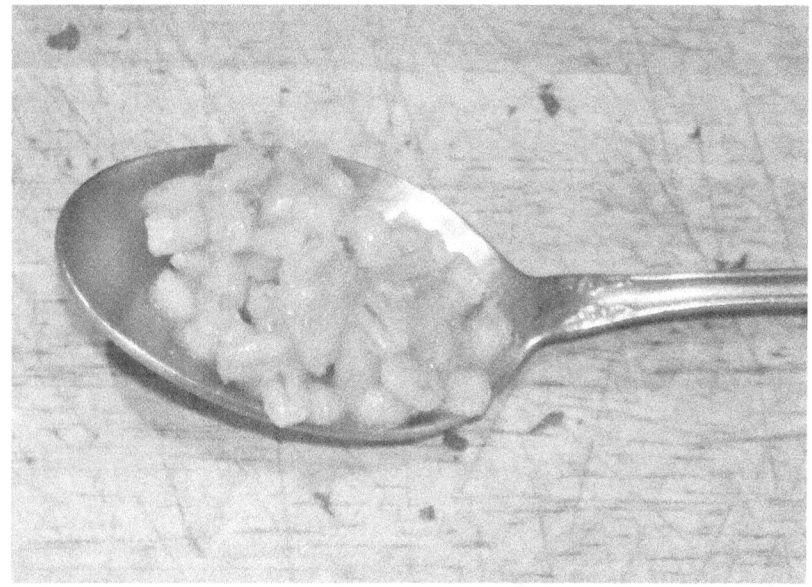

Take the pan from the heat and stir in the cooked tomatoes, chopped parsley, chopped thyme, chopped basil and the grated Parmesan. Add the rest of the salt and pepper and stir the mixture so that everything is combined.

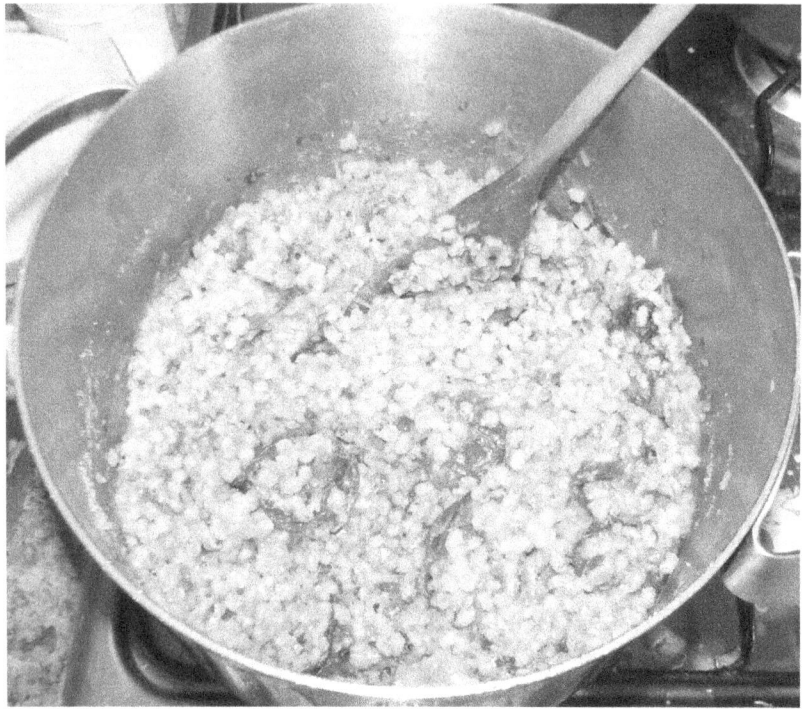

Put the risotto into a serving bowl and garnish with the baked tomatoes, basil leaves and more grated Parmesan. Serve immediately while nice and hot.

Humus

Humus is a classic Mediterranean dish full of good honest tasty ingredients which will all add to your Mediterranean diet. Serve it with Wholemeal Pita bread and you then have it all. There is a recipe for making your own tahini which means that you can cut down on shop made ingredients and use your own extra virgin olive oil to make it with.

You can easily make your own homemade humus using this simple recipe. With a recipe this simple and tasty you won't want to go back to shop bought humus ever again.

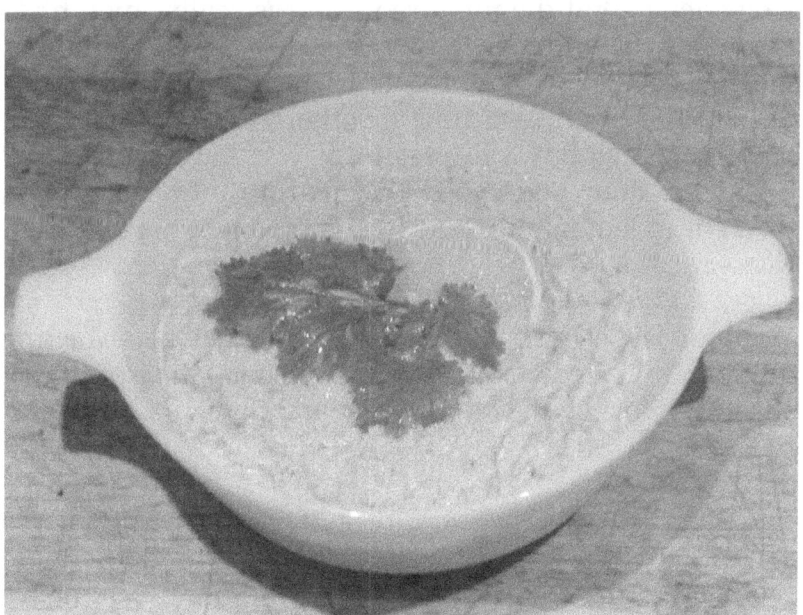

Humus with coriander

Ingredients

400g can chickpeas
1 tbsp tahini paste
1 large garlic clove
3 tbsp Greek style yogurt
Lemon juice
Salt and pepper

Method

Chop the large garlic clove. You need both the chickpeas and the liquid from the can of chickpeas so open the can and drain the liquid through a sieve into a small bowl.

Put the yogurt, chickpeas, tahini and chopped garlic into a blender. Blend the mixture until it is really smooth. At this point the humus will be really thick so add a little of the saved chickpea liquid and blend again. Only add a little of the liquid at a time or otherwise the humus will become too sloppy. Repeat until you have the desired thickness. Pour and spoon the mixture into a bowl and then stir in lemon juice and seasoning to get the taste that you want.

You can leave out the tahini and still get good tasting humus. Half a teaspoon of cumin powder can also act as a substitute for the flavour of the tahini if you haven't got it to hand.

You can also experiment with adding other ingredients such as fresh coriander leaves, cumin, paprika, roasted red peppers or ground chilli. If you find that the humus is a little bitter then you should consider cutting back on the amount of tahini paste. You can also substitute lime for lemon which will give the recipe an extra dimension.

If you find getting the tahini paste a difficulty you can make your own by blending 3 parts sesame seeds with 1 part olive oil. As well as being homemade it can also cut down the cost of buying the tahini paste.

You can make a spicy harissa topping for the humus by mixing 2 tbsp of harissa paste with 1 tbsp of tomato puree.

You can also prepare your own chickpeas from uncooked ones. This does take a lot longer to do but home prepared chickpeas tend to be a lot softer than the canned ones and as a result they can end up making a more buttery and smooth humus.

To prepare your own chickpeas you should first put 200g of the uncooked chickpeas in a bowl. Next add twice the volume of cold water to cover them. Mix in 1 teaspoon of bicarbonate of soda and then leave the chickpeas to soak for 24 hours. After this time, drain the water from the chickpeas and rinse them well in cold water. Add the chickpeas to a large saucepan and add ½ a teaspoon of bicarbonate of soda. Cover the pan and then heat until boiling. Reduce the heat and simmer for between 1 and 2 hours. If the water level drops add more boiling water to the pan during cooking. After cooking leave the pan to cool and then drain the chickpeas well making sure that you save the cooking water from the pan for use later. These cooked chickpeas can be used in the humus recipe in the same way as the canned ones and the cooking water used as before to get the right consistency for the humus. If you prepare a lot of cooked chickpeas you can freeze them in portions for use in later humus recipes.

Mediterranean Diet Exercise

Exercise is an important part of the Mediterranean lifestyle which can help to increase the health of your heart. As detailed in the previous chapters, the local people of the Mediterranean regions get their exercise by having to do such things as walking up hills, physical work in their garden and also any odd jobs that they might end up doing. The life could be considered hard and as a result exercise is what you have to do to survive. It isn't something that you do by choice in order to make yourself healthy. In the rest of the world we all have the choice to do exercise but most of us fail to act on that choice. Often we do things such as joining a gym but then follow this up by not going. It is as if the act of suffering by paying for the gym is in fact a substitute for actually going there! Exercise is all around us we just have to engage in it. It often doesn't cost anything to actually do it.

Walking

The easiest way to start getting your exercise is to take up some form of walking. You should think about the journeys that you make. Which of those could you actually do by walking instead of using the car? Local shopping is the obvious choice. Make a decision to walk to the shops rather than driving there. Where I live the shops are about half a mile away in the village centre. This is about 3 minutes in the car and 10 minutes walking. When I go by car I have to pay for the petrol and then find somewhere to park the car. This means that I don't really save that much time compared to walking there. We always say that we don't have the time to spare and that therefore we have to use the car. In this example there is little difference time wise. I choose to walk when I can. Obviously I sometimes get put off if the weather is bad but how many times is it going to be that bad that walking is not a suitable choice? Walking there and back is therefore a 20 minute exercise. During the day I could do this to fetch my morning paper, go to the bakery and go to the bank. Obviously I could do this all in one trip but by splitting up the tasks into individual trips and spreading them out through the day I get three times the amount of exercise and this then can soon mount up to an hour in the end.

When you do walking it is good if you can raise your pulse rate for part of the journey. This could be achieved by walking faster for part of the time or by walking up hills. There are 2 routes that I use to walk to my local shops. The one is flat and the other goes through the park and up a hill. As a result when I do the out journey I tend to walk along the flat route and do part of it quickly. This then raises my pulse rate during the quick part. On my return journey I go through the park and up the hill. The hill is quite steep and as a result once again I manage to increase my pulse rate. You too can set up some regular short walks that can do the same by simply planning where you go and the routes that you can take. Walking when you have a purpose is a good way of making sure that it gets done. I walk to the library to change my son's books. I walk to the local bar to see my friends. All of these walking trips add to the amounts of exercise that I do on a regular basis. You can also consider walking to work, if your work place is relatively near to where you live. I used to walk from my house to the centre of the city where my work was located. This was a journey of about 40 minutes and involved having to walk up a really steep hill. Walking to work not only gave me over an hour of valuable exercise each day but also saved me money in petrol and parking for the car. In addition to this I also had a wonderful walk back along a beautiful water way. It is unfortunate that work these days isn't near by and as a result I miss out on this valuable source of exercise. However, all is not lost because; I have traded this walk to work for another shorter one where I walk my son to and from his school each day.

Some people enjoy longer walking sessions for pleasure as well as exercise. Walking is a good way to explore a new area or to take in some wonderful local scenery. These walks tend to be longer and will need planning. You can get books showing popular local walks and there may even be a section is your local newspaper which will gives maps of interesting walks to go on. These walks don't have to be just in your local area. You can drive to a new area and then do a planned walk for an hour or two. These types of walk can be very enjoyable and they can be a good way of spending leisure time. You can make these walks more enjoyable if you take a friend or a group of friends with you. As we are social creatures, having company can really encourage us to do more and more walking. If your friends aren't up for joining in with your new walking activities you could consider joining a regular walking group such as the 'Ramblers'. My mother did this and she got a lot of enjoyment from going on walks and rambles with her group. This was as much a social activity as a type of exercise. As with all types of exercise you should make sure that you start your new walking activity slowly and steadily. Don't be tempted to start off with really long walks, really fast walking, or walking up really steep long hills. Take things easy to start off with, and then gradually stretch yourself until you reach an activity level that you are happy with.

Cycling

Cycling is another way of getting exercise. You can get the mountain bike out of the garage that you haven't used for a few years now. Cycling has the benefit of enabling you to increase your pulse rate and make your heart work harder in quite a short amount of time. Making your heart do some work is a good thing. It keeps it fit and healthy and ready to take on the pressures of life when it has to. Without keeping your heart fit and healthy you could find that it gives out on you when you need it next time to run for the bus or other sudden activities. Once again you should start off slowly and gradually build up a routine for using your bike. There are often bike dedicated paths these days and using these can help to keep you safe as you minimize your exposure to dangerous traffic. There is one such cycle path near to where I live and I use it a lot. There is a café someway along the track and this gives me an incentive to get on my bike and go there. It is a kind of reward. I also have my coffee of the day at the café which means that I am following the aims of my Mediterranean diet. Cycling also allows you to get to more places when you compare it to walking. This in turn can make life interesting and make you want to keep your cycling activities going.

Gardening

Gardening is one of the pastimes that the Greek islanders did in order to keep fit and there is no reason why you shouldn't engage in this yourself. There are plenty of activities in gardening which will manage to get your pulse racing a little. There is the digging to start off with. This involves a lot of hard work and once again you should work up to it by doing a little to start off with and stretching yourself a little more each time you do it. You should also take care that you are doing your digging correctly as you could end up with back problems, if you aren't careful. Then there is all of the fetching, carrying, cutting and planting involved in gardening. This is also valuable exercise. In the summer months there is a lot of grass mowing to do and I certainly get my exercise a few times each week when I have to push the lawnmower over the front and back lawns of my house.

Gardening can also have its rewards. This can involve the creation of a beautiful and pleasing environment around you and a sense of achievement. A sense of well being goes a long way to making you feel healthy. A happy mind can help to keep your body healthy as well. Another benefit of doing some gardening is that you can grow your own fresh vegetables and herbs. This in turn will cut down your costs as well as providing the freshest foods that you can get. You can also make sure that your fresh greens are free of pesticides and other chemicals by not using them on your crops.

Starting a garden will involve some planning and you will have to do more than just think about it because Spring quickly comes and goes, and before long you may have missed the growing season before you have finished your procrastination. As with all things in life, you have to act and actually do something about it. If you don't have a garden yourself you may find that your local authority may provide areas of land that you can rent from them in order to grow your own plants. These are called allotments and because they are often situated in a group you can actually make friends with like minded people, exchange ideas and get help if you come across problems when you are trying to grow your plants.

Sport

Another idea to get involved in exercise is to take up a sport that you once may have done when you were younger. There are plenty of sporting clubs that will allow you to take up activities such as tennis, bowling, cricket, badminton and even such things as rock climbing. I have noticed that a lot of my friends have taken up golf. This is not a bad thing to do because you can go and play with friends and get your exercise walking the links and playing the ball. This again, is another social activity that will add to the richness of your life. Some friends of mine recently took up archery. They are already addicted to it, have their own bows and attend their archery club every weekend. The one of them is looking to buy a long bow and even make his own arrows. There are plenty of sports that you can take up and plenty of clubs that will be more than happy to let you join them. I prefer to do things on my own or with the family so a little mountain biking down local tracks with my son is ideal. Sport can be fun, and as a result it is well worth thinking about getting involved and adding this as an exercise to complement your Mediterranean diet.

Conclusion

This book shows that there is mounting evidence for the health benefits of following a Mediterranean style diet. A lot of doctors have been recommending it to their patients for many years, despite the lack of real scientific studies. After the latest Spanish study there really isn't any doubt any more. It is time to evaluate your own diet and change your lifestyle and diet for the sake of your heart.

The big problem that a lot of people have is how to follow such a diet when you don't actually live on the sunny shores of the Mediterranean and don't have a rural rustic life. The people on the Greek island of Ikaria are practically forced to follow their lifestyle by the conditions under which they live. In the rest of the world there are so many distractions that it becomes very difficult to follow a diet different to the rest of the local population. This book offers some good advice about how you can make changes to your own diet so that it will follow the principles central to the Mediterranean diet. This will then have great benefits for you heart and general health. The basic idea is that you should slowly change things by eliminating the bad foods and including the good ones. In this way the whole thing won't come as a total shock.

The Mediterranean diet is also about exercise and as a result you should take the advice in the book and try to increase the amount of exercise that you do. As suggested you can get extra exercise by using the car less and also taking up a sport that you once may have done while you were younger. The important thing is to try and allow time for some exercise. We all lead busy lives and time seems to be of the utmost importance. However, when you take an overview of your time you should see that we worry too much about unimportant things that get in the way of us being able to do the things that we want to.

This book includes a selection of recipes that you can start to include in your regular meals. They are vegetarian and fish based and hardly include any meat elements at all. The amount of dairy product is also much reduced. You may like to search for further recipes but you should make sure that they are actual Mediterranean ones rather than some trendy Chef's interpretation of a meal from this region. You can also adapt recipes so that they are more like Mediterranean ones. This may involve changing the oil used to Olive oil, reducing the amounts of dairy product used or restricting the amount of meat that they contain.

One further good idea is to have a holiday in the Mediterranean region and try to eat the local cuisine rather than that served up for the tourists. This may involve travelling to more out of the way places but this in itself will make your holiday more interesting and entertaining. Experiencing the things that people actually do eat in the Mediterranean will give you a welcome boost to your confidence and allow you to be more adventurous with your cooking once you return home.

About the Author

Elisabetta Parisi has written several other books specializing in various recipes from different European countries including her home country Italy. Here are the details of some of the other books that you can buy.

Making your own pasta is a very satisfying way to spend your time in the kitchen. The rewards come from both the effort that you put in and the fantastic new tastes that you can create for your family and friends at meal time.

Homemade Pasta Dough explains how to make many different kinds of pasta from the raw ingredients. The book explains how to make pasta dough both by hand and using various machines to help cut down the work involved.

Fresh pasta made at home is a very healthy option and there are lots of ways that you can vary the pasta dough you make. This will then add life to your pasta meals. The book contains details of mixing, rolling, cutting, stuffing and shaping your pasta.

This is an updated and extended version of the original popular book with lots of new pasta dough recipes which will extend your pasta repertoire. There are also more details on stuffed pastas such as ravioli and tortellini as well as dessert style pasta. Also now included, are example recipes showing where the different pasta doughs and shapes can be used.

http://www.amazon.com/Homemade-Pasta-Dough-including-ravioli/dp/147823458X

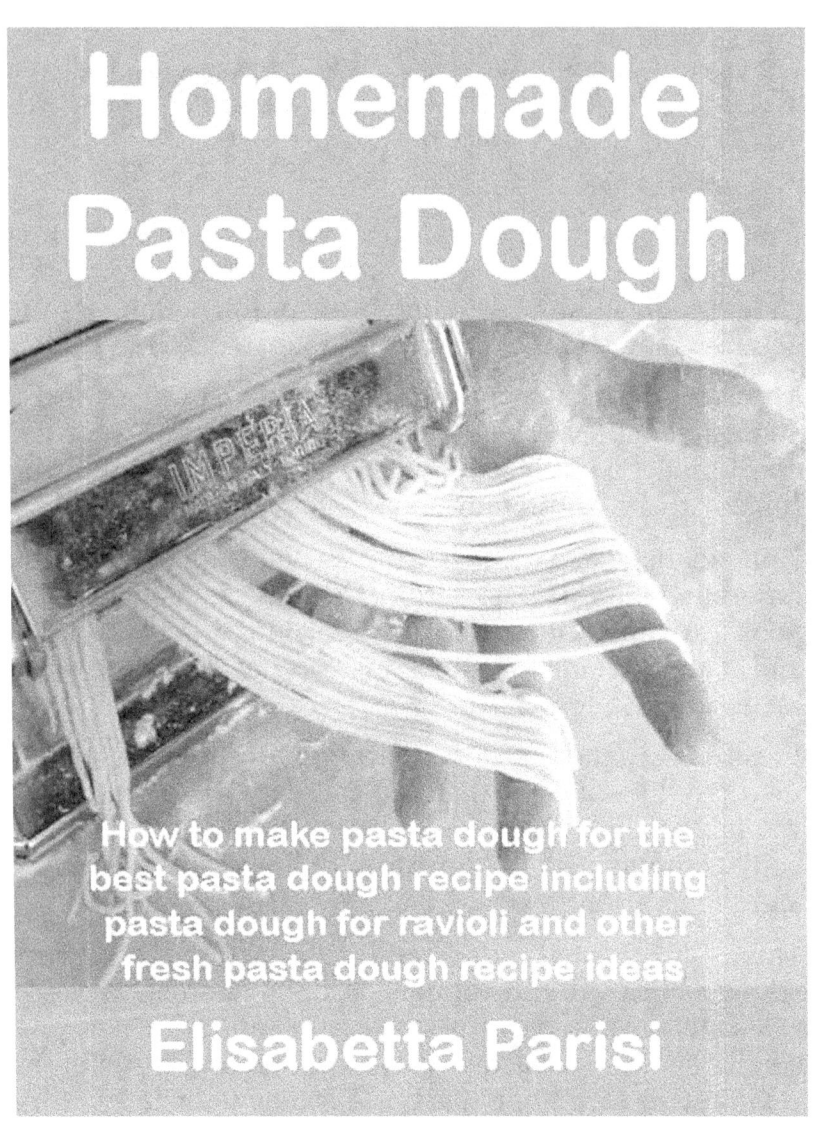

Homemade Pasta Dough

How to make pasta dough for the best pasta dough recipe including pasta dough for ravioli and other fresh pasta dough recipe ideas

Elisabetta Parisi

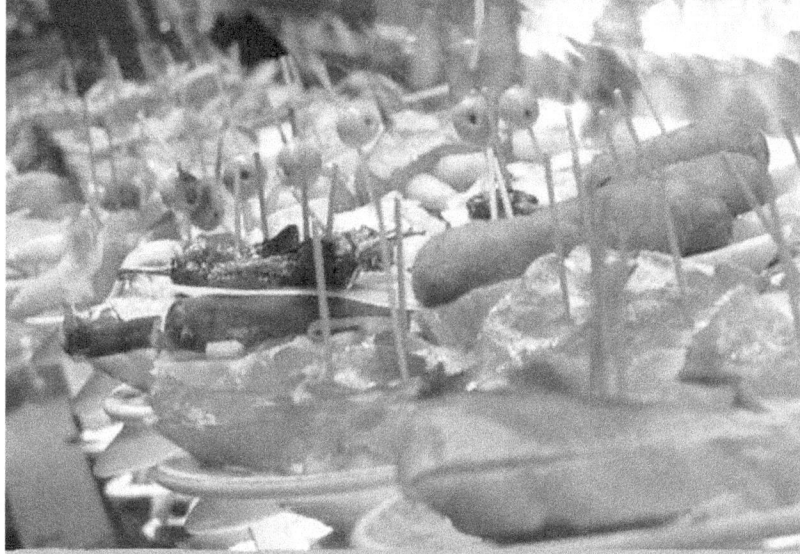

Tapas Recipes

Covers what are tapas and includes Spanish tapas recipes to make lots of tapas dishes so that you can build your own tapas menu based on Spanish tapas and other world tapas ideas

Elisabetta Parisi

http://www.amazon.com/Tapas-Recipes-Spanish-recipes-ebook/dp/B005KLTCEY

Tapas Recipes has lots of tasty tapas foods for you to make at home. Tapas food is becoming more popular all of the time with tapas bars opening up across the world and big supermarkets stocking their own tapas lines. You can make your own tapas out of fresh ingredients, enjoy them with some Spanish wine and relive those glorious summer holiday times. Tapas are great as snacks and even better with wine or beer. They are also a great alternative to the usual sausage rolls and paste sandwiches of a typical buffet spread. Enjoy them on your own and contemplate the world or entertain with them it is your choice! Each recipe is easy to follow with no strange ingredients that are hard to get. Go on, have a change and make some tapas.

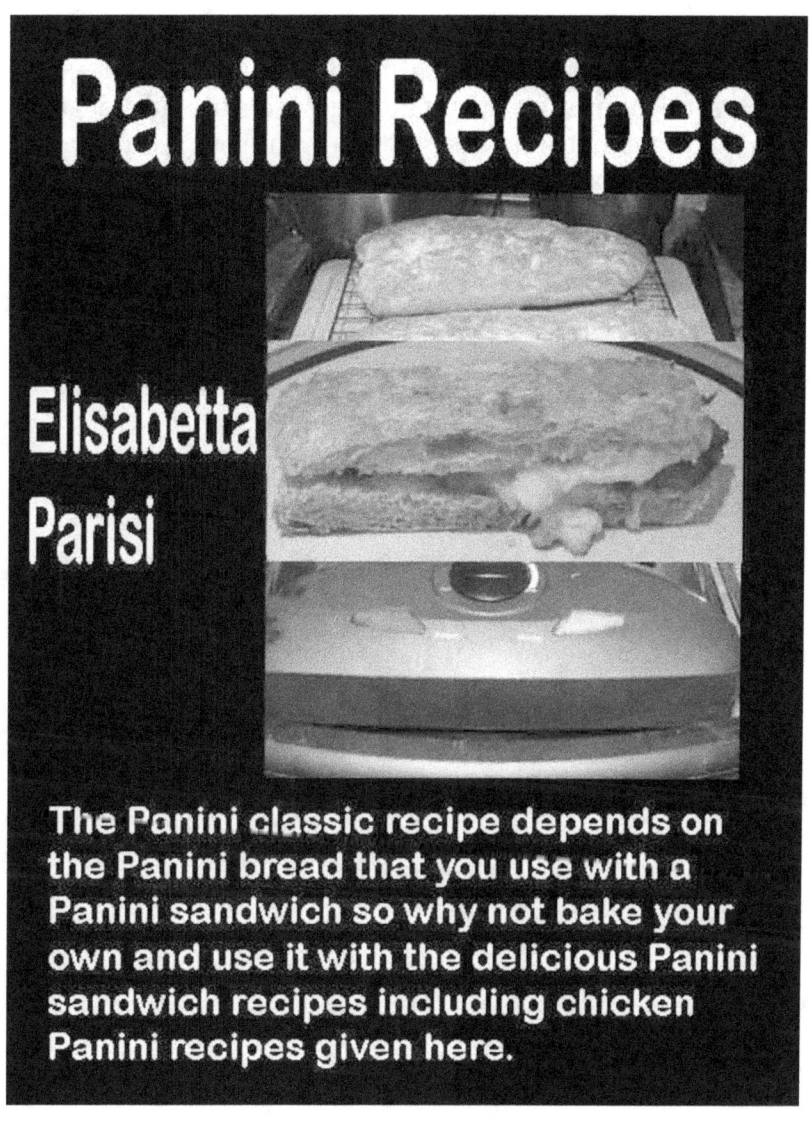

Panini Recipes

Elisabetta Parisi

The Panini classic recipe depends on the Panini bread that you use with a Panini sandwich so why not bake your own and use it with the delicious Panini sandwich recipes including chicken Panini recipes given here.

http://www.amazon.com/Panini-Recipes-sandwich-including-ebook/dp/B005F5GPHM

Panini Recipes can be exciting as well as quick. You are really missing out if you don't have this Italian inspired food at home. You can put just about anything into a panini so long as it is cooked first. The taste of a panini is influenced by the quality of the bread that you use. You can buy Italian bread but why not go that extra step and make some yourself. This book contains some easy recipes for panini bread including Ciabatta and Focaccia. You can make these quickly and improve your panini experience greatly. Try your new homemade panini bread with some of the exciting panini recipes in this book.

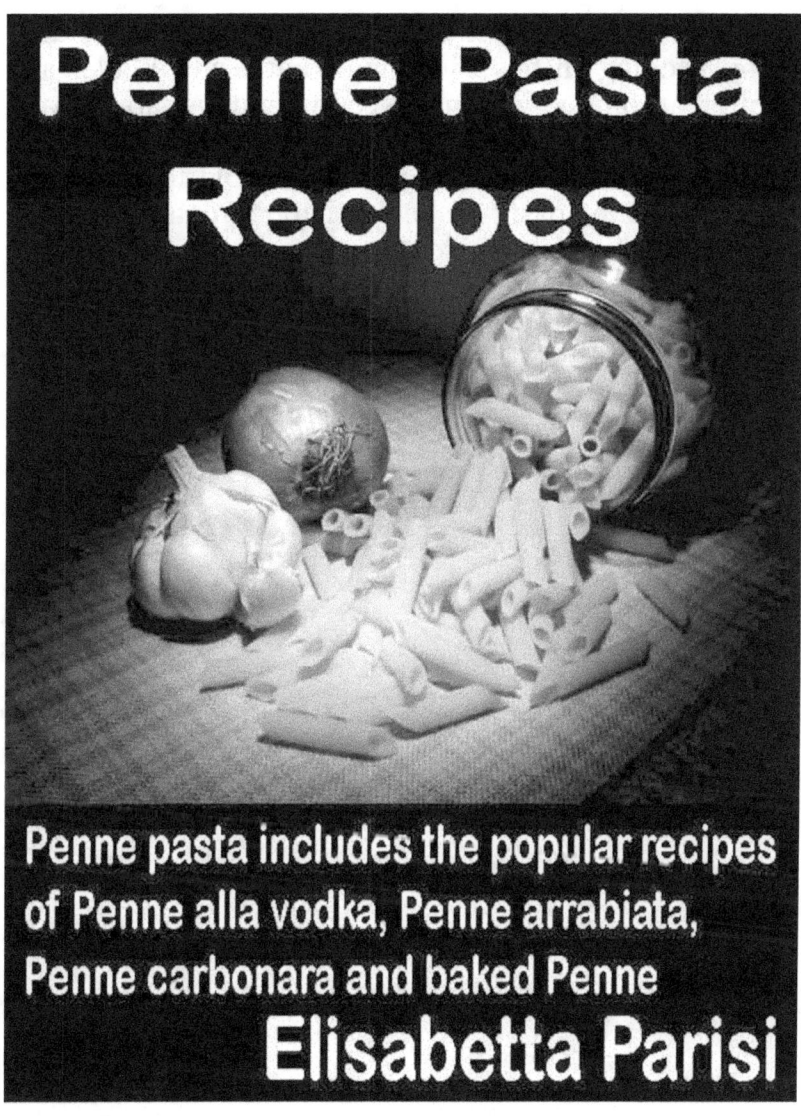

Penne pasta includes the popular recipes of Penne alla vodka, Penne arrabiata, Penne carbonara and baked Penne

Elisabetta Parisi

http://www.amazon.com/Penne-Pasta-Recipes-arrabiata-ebook/dp/B005JL4PWE

Penne Pasta Recipes for great meals using this very versatile pasta shape. Penne is fantastic with sauces, in soups and with salads. Learn how to cook Penne so that it can absorb and hold the sauces you add to it. Make the basic Marinara sauce and you can use this as the basis for a lot of other recipes and build upon its flavors to produce many exciting dishes including Penne alla Vodka and Penne Carbonara. Feel the spice in Penne Arrabiatta and cook with Italian sausage for extra flavor. Learn the recipes in this book and you will be able to produce a huge variety of pasta dishes rather than the inevitable Spag Bol which seems to turn up on the menu every week.

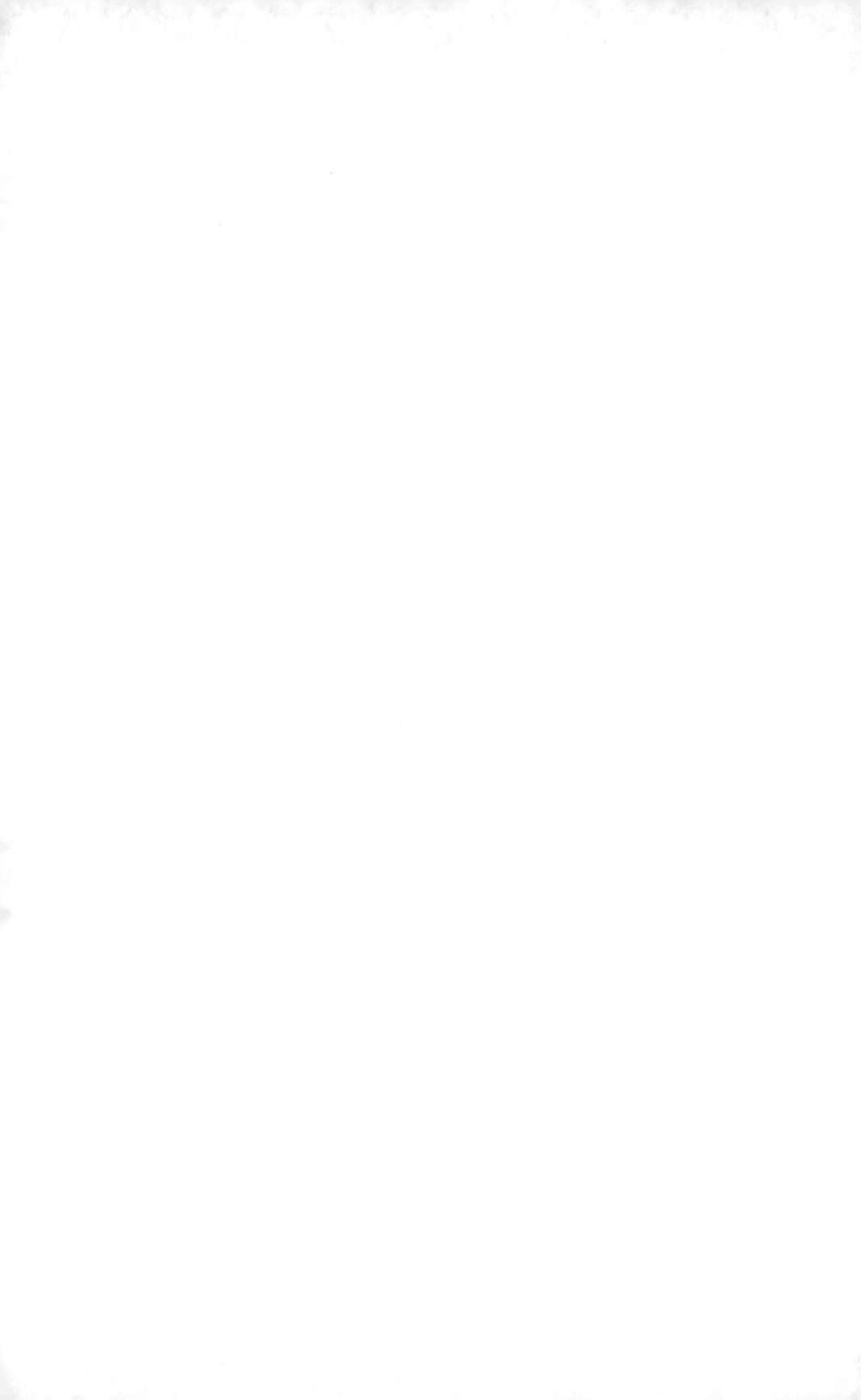